STATISTICS APPLIED TO CLINICAL TRIALS
SECOND EDITION

Statistics Applied to Clinical Trials,
Second Edition

by

TON J. CLEOPHAS, MD, PhD, Associate-Professor,
President American College of Angiology,
Co-Chair Module Statistics Applied tot Clinical Trials,
European Interuniversity College of Pharmaceutical Medicine Lyon, France,
Internist-clinical pharmacologist,
Department Medicine, Albert Schweitzer Hospital, Dordrecht, The Netherlands

AEILKO H. ZWINDERMAN, Math D, PhD, Professor,
Co-Chair Module Statistics Applied to Clinical Trials,
European Interuniversity College of Pharmaceutical Medicine Lyon, France,
Professor of Statistics,
Department Biostatistics and Epidemiology, Academic Medical Center Amsterdam,
The Netherlands

and

TOINE F. CLEOPHAS, D Techn,
Technical University, Delft, The Netherlands

Kluwer Academic Publishers
Dordrecht / Boston / London

A C.I.P. Catalogue record for this book is available from the Library of Congress.

ISBN 1-4020-0569-5

Published by Kluwer Academic Publishers,
P.O. Box 17, 3300 AA Dordrecht, The Netherlands.

Sold and distributed in North, Central and South America
by Kluwer Academic Publishers,
101 Philip Drive, Norwell, MA 02061, U.S.A.

In all other countries, sold and distributed
by Kluwer Academic Publishers,
P.O. Box 322, 3300 AH Dordrecht, The Netherlands.

Printed on acid-free paper

Printed in the Netherlands.

TABLE OF CONTENTS

PREFACE

The European Interuniversity Diploma of Pharmaceutical Medicine is a postacademic course of 2-3 years sponsored by the Socrates program of the European Community. The office of this interuniversity project is in Lyon and the lectures are given there. The European Community has provided a building and will remunerate lecturers. The institute which provides the teaching is called the European College of Pharmaceutical Medicine, and is affiliated with 15 universities throughout Europe, whose representatives constitute the academic committee. This committee supervises educational objectives. Start lectures February 2000.

There are about 20 modules for the first two years of training, most of which are concerned with typically pharmacological and clinical pharmacological matters including pharmacokinetics, pharmacodynamics, phase III clinical trials, reporting, communication, ethics and, any other aspects of drug development. Subsequent training consists of practice training within clinical research organisations, universities, regulatory bodies etc., and finally of a dissertation. The diploma, and degree are delivered by the Claude Bernard University in Lyon as well as the other participating universities.

The module "Statistics applied to clinical trials" wil be taught in the form of a 3 to 6 day yearly course given in Lyon and starting February 2000. Lecturers have to submit a document of the course (this material will be made available to students). Three or 4 lecturers are requested to prepare detailed written material for students as well as to prepare examination of the students. The module is thus an inportant part of a postgraduate course for physicians and pharmacists for the purpose of obtaining the European diploma of pharmaceutical medicine. The diploma should make for leading positions in pharmaceutical industry, academic drug research, as well as regulatory bodies within the EC. This module is mainly involved in the statistics of randomized clinical trials .

The chapters 1-9, 11, 17, 18 of this book are based on the module "Medical statistics applied to clinical trials" and contain material that should be mastered by the students before their exams. The remaining chapters are capita selecta intended for excellent students and are not included in the exams.

The authors believe that this book is innovative in the statistical literature because, unlike most introductory books in medical statistics, it provides an explanatory rather than mathematical approach to statistics, and, in addition, emphasizes non-classical but increasingly frequently used methods for the statistical analyses of clinical trials, e.g., equivalence testing, sequential analyses, multiple linear regression analyses for confounding, interaction, and synergism.The authors are not aware of any other work published so far that is comparable with the current work, and, therefore, believe that it does fill a need.

August 1999
Dordrecht, Leiden , Delft

PREFACE TO SECOND EDITION

In this second edition the authors have removed textual errors from the first edition. Also seven new chapters (chapters 8, 10, 13, 15-18) have been added. The principles of regression analysis and its resemblance to analysis of variance was missing in the first edition, and have been described in chapter 8. Chapter 10 assesses curvilinear regression. Chapter 13 describes the statistical analyses of crossover data with binary response. The latest developments including statistical analyses of genetic data and quality-of-life data have been described in chapters 15 and 16. Emphasis is given in chapters 17 and 18 to the limitations of statistics to assess non-normal data, and to the similarities between commonly-used statistical tests. Finally, additional tables including the Mann-Whitney and Wilcoxon rank sum tables have been added in the Appendix.

December 2001
Dordrecht, Amsterdam, Delft

FOREWORD

In clinical medicine appropriate statistics has become indispensable to evaluate treatment effects. Randomized controlled trials are currently the only trials that truly provide evidence-based medicine. Evidence based medicine has become crucial to optimal treatment of patients. We can define randomized controlled trials by using Christopher J. Bulpitt's definition "a carefully and ethically designed experiment which includes the provision of adequate and appropriate controls by a process of randomization, so that precisely framed questions can be answered". The answers given by randomized controlled trials constitute at present the way how patients should be clinically managed. In the setup of such randomized trial one of the most important issues is the statistical basis. The randomized trial will never work when the statistical grounds and analyses have not been clearly defined beforehand. All endpoints should be clearly defined in order to perform appropriate power calculations. Based on these power calculations the exact number of available patients can be calculated in order to have a sufficient quantity of individuals to have the predefined questions answered. Therefore, every clinical physician should be capable to understand the statistical basis of well performed clinical trials. It is therefore a great pleasure that Drs. T.J.Cleophas, A.H.Zwinderman, and T.F. Cleophas have published a book on statistical analysis of clinical trials. The book entitled "Statistics Applied to Clinical Trials"is clearly written and makes complex issues in statistical analysis transparant. Apart from providing the classical issues in statistical analysis, the authors also address novel issues such as interim analyses, sequential analyses, and meta-analyses. The book is composed of 18 chapters, which are nicely structured. The authors have deepened our insight in the applications of statistical analysis of clinical trials. We would like to congratulate the editors on this achievement and hope that many readers will enjoy reading this intriguing book.

E.E. van der Wall, MD, PhD, Professor of Cardiology, President Netherlands Association of Cardiology, Leiden, Netherlands

CHAPTER 1

HYPOTHESES, DATA, STRATIFICATION

1. GENERAL CONSIDERATIONS

Over the past decades the randomized clinical trial has entered an era of continuous improvement and has gradually become accepted as the most effective way of determining the relative efficacy and toxicity of new drug therapies. This course is mainly involved in the methods of prospective randomized clinical trials of new drugs. Other methods for assessment including open-evaluation-studies, cohort- and case-control studies, although sometimes used, e.g., for pilot studies and for the evaluation of long term drug-effects, are excluded in this course. Traditionally, clinical drug trials are divided into IV phases (from phase I for initial testing to phase IV after release for general use), but scientific rules governing different phases are very much the same, and can thus be discussed simultaneously.

A. CLEARLY DEFINED HYPOTHESES

Hypotheses must be tested prospectively with hard data, and against placebo or known forms of therapies that are in place and considered to be effective. Uncontrolled studies won't succeed to give a definitive answer if they are ever so clever. Uncontrolled studies while of value in the absence of scientific controlled studies, their conclusions represent merely suggestions and hypotheses. The scientific method requires to look at some controls to characterize the defined population.

B. VALID DESIGNS

Any research but certainly industrially sponsored drug research where sponsors benefit from favorable results, benefits from valid designs. A valid study means a study unlikely to be biased, or unlikely to include systematic errors. The most dangerous error in clinical trials are systematic errors otherwise called biases. Validity is the most important thing for doers of clinical trials to check. Trials should be made independent, objective, balanced, blinded, controlled, with objective measurements, with adequate sample sizes to test the expected treatment effects, with random assignment of patients.

C. EXPLICIT DESCRIPTION OF METHODS

Explicit description of the methods should include description of the recruitment procedures, method of randomization of the patients, prior statements about the methods of assessments of generating and analysis of the data and the statistical methods used, accurate ethics including written informed consent.

D. UNIFORM DATA ANALYSIS

Uniform and appropriate data analysis generally starts with plots or tables of actual data.

Statistics then comes in to test primary hypotheses primarily. Data that do not answer prior hypotheses may be tested for robustness or sensitivity, otherwise called precision of point estimates e.g., dependent upon numbers of outliers. The results of studies with many outliers and thus little precision should be interpreted with caution. It is common practice for studies to test multiple measurements for the purpose of answering one single question, e.g., the benefit to health of a new drug may be estimated by mortality in addition to various morbidity variables, and there is nothing wrong with that practice. We should not make any formal correction for multiple comparisons of this kind. Instead, we should informally integrate all the data before reaching conclusions, and look for the trends without judging one or two low P-values among otherwise high P-values as proof.

However, subgroup analyses involving post-hoc comparisons by dividing the data into groups with different ages, prior conditions, gender etc can easily generate hundreds of P values. If investigators test many different hypotheses, they are apt to find significant differences at least 5% of the time. To make sense of this kind of results, we need to consider the Bonferroni inequality, which will be emphasized in chapter 9, and states that if k statistical tests are performed with the cutoff level for a test statistic, for example t or F, at the α level, the likelihood for observing a value of the test statistic exceeding the cutoff level is no greater than k times α. For example, if we wish to do three comparisons with t-tests while keeping the probability of making a mistake less than 5%, we use instead of $\alpha=5\%$ in this case $\alpha=5/3\%=1.6\%$. With many more tests, analyses soon lose any sensitivity and do hardly prove anything anymore. Nonetheless a limited number of post-hoc analyses, particularly when a plausible theory is underlying, can be useful in generating hypotheses for future studies.

2. TWO MAIN HYPOTHESES IN DRUG TRIALS: EFFICACY AND SAFETY

Drug trials are mainly for addressing the efficacy as well as the safety of the drugs to be tested in them. For analyzing efficacy data formal statistical techniques are normally used. Basically, the null hypothesis of no treatment effect is tested, and is rejected when difference from zero is significant. For such purpose a great variety of statistical significance tests has been developed, all of whom report P values, and compute confidence intervals to estimate the magnitude of the treatment effect. The appropriate test depends upon the type of data and will be discussed in the next chapter. Of safety data, such as adverse events, data are mostly collected with the hope of demonstrating that the test treatment is not different from control. This concept is based upon a different hypothesis from that proposed for efficacy data, where the very objective is generally to show that there actually is a difference between test and control. Because the objective of collecting safety data is thus different, the approach to analysis must be likewise different. In particular, it may be less appropriate to use statistical significance tests to analyze the latter data. A significance test is a tool that can help to establish whether a difference between treatments is likely to be real. It cannot be used to demonstrate that two treatments are similar in their effects. In addition, safety data, more frequently than efficacy data, consist of proportions and percentages rather than continuous data as will be discussed in the next section. Usually, the best approach to analysis of these kinds of data is to present suitable summary statistics, together with confidence intervals. In the case of adverse event data, the rate of occurrence of each distinct adverse event on each treatment group should be reported, together with confidence intervals for the difference between the rates of occurrence on the different treatments. An alternative would be to present risk ratios or relative risks of occurrence, with confidence intervals for the relative risk. Chapter 3 mainly addresses the analyses of these kinds of data.

Other aspects of assessing similarity rather than difference between treatments will be discussed separately in chapter 6 where the theory, equations, and assessments are given for demonstrating statistical equivalence.

3. DIFFERENT TYPES OF DATA: CONTINUOUS DATA

The first step, before any analysis or plotting of data can be performed, is to decide what kind of data we have. Usually data are continuous, e.g., blood pressures, heart rates etc. But regularly proportions or percentages are used for the assessment of part of the data. The next few lines will address how we can summarize and characterize these two different approaches to the data.

Samples of **continuous data** are characterized by

$$\textbf{Mean} = \Sigma \textbf{x} \ /\textbf{n} \ ,$$

where Σ is the summation, x are the individual data and n is the total number of data.

$$\textbf{Variance between the data} = \Sigma \ (\ \textbf{x} - \bar{x} \ )^2 \ / \ \textbf{(n-1)}$$

$$\textbf{Standard deviation (SD)} = \sqrt{} \ \textbf{(Variance)}$$

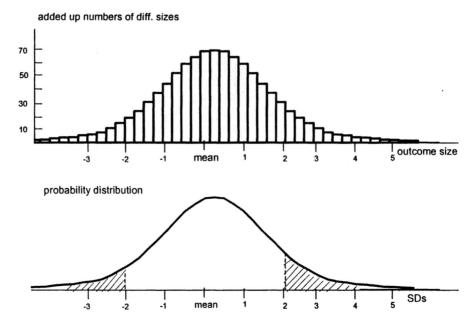

Figure 1. Histogram and Gaussian curve representation of data.

Continuous data can be plotted in the form of a histogram (Figure 1 upper graph). On the x-axis, frequently called z-axis in statistics, it has individual data. On the y-axis it has "how often". For example, the mean value is observed most frequently, while the bars on either side gradually grow shorter. This graph adequately represents the data. It is, however, not adequate for statistical analyses. Figure 1 lower graph pictures a Gaussian curve, otherwise called normal (distribution) curve. On the x-axis we have, again, the individual data, expressed either in absolute data or in SDs distant from the mean. On the y-axis the bars have been replaced with a continuous line. It is now impossible to determine from the graph how many patients had a particular outcome. Instead, important inferences can be made. For example, the total area under the curve (AUC) represents 100% of the data, AUC left from mean represents 50% of the data, left from -1 SDs it has 15.87% of the data, left from -2SDs it has 2.5% of the data. This graph is better for statistical purposes but not yet good enough.

Figure 2 gives two Gaussian curves, a narrow and a wide one. Both are based on

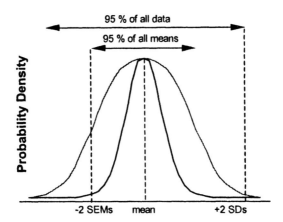

Figure 2. Two examples of normal distributions.

the same data, but with different meaning. The wide one sumarizes the data of our trial. The narrow one sumarizes the mean of many trials similar to our trial. We won't try to make you understand why this is so. Still, it is easy to conceive that the distribution of all means of many trials is narrower and has fewer outliers than the distribution of the actual data from our trial, and that it will center around the mean of our trial because out trial is assumed to be representative for the entire population. You may find it hard to believe but the narrow curve with standard errors of the mean (SEMs) or simply SEs on the x-axis can be effectively used for testing important statistical hypotheses, like (1) no difference between new and standard treatment, (2) a real difference, (3) the new treatment is better than the standard treatment, (4) the two treatments equivalent. Thus, mean ± 2 SDs (or more precisely 1.96 SDs) represents the AUC of the wide distribution, otherwise called the 95% confidence interval of the data, which means that 95 % of the data of the sample are within. The SEM-curve (narrow one) is narrower than the SD-curve (wide one) because SEM= SD/√n. Mean ± 2 sems (or more precisely 1.96 SEMs) represents 95% of the means of many trials similar to our trial.

$$SEM= SD / \sqrt{n}$$

As the size of SEM in the graph is about 1/3 times SD, the number of each sample is here about 10. The area under the narrow curve represents 100 % of the means we would obtain, while the area under the curve of the wide graph represents 100% of all of the data of the samples.

Why is this SEM approach so important in statistics. Statistics makes use of mean values and their standard error to test the null hypotheses of finding in your sample no difference from zero. When we reject a null hypothesis at P<0.05 it literally means that there is < 5 % chance that the mean value of our sample crosses the area of the null hypothesis where we say there is no difference. It does not mean that many individual data may not be beyond that boundary. So, actually it is just a matter of agreement. But it works well.

So remember:
Mean ± 2 SDs covers an area under the curve including 95 % of the data of the given sample.
Mean ± 2 SEMs covers an area under curve including 95% of the means of many samples.

In statistical analysis we often compare different samples by taking their sums or differences. Again, this text is not intended to explain the procedures but results can be used even so.

The distributions of the sums as well as those of the difference of samples are again normal distributions and can be characterized by

$$\text{Sum: } \textbf{mean}_1 + \textbf{mean}_2 \pm \sqrt{(\textbf{SD}_1^2 + \textbf{SD}_2^2)}$$

$$\text{Difference: } \textbf{mean}_1 - \textbf{mean}_2 \pm \sqrt{(\textbf{SD}_1^2 + \textbf{SD}_2^2)}$$

$$\text{if } n_1 = n_2 = n$$

$$\textbf{SEM}_{sum} = \sqrt{(\textbf{SD}_1^2 / n + \textbf{SD}_1^2 / n)}$$

$$\textbf{SEM}_{difference} = \qquad \text{``}$$

Note: if if $n_1 \neq n_2$

$$\sqrt{(\textbf{SD}_1^2 + \textbf{SD}_2^2)} \text{ turns into } \sqrt{(n_1 \textbf{SD}_1^2 + n_2 \textbf{SD}_2^2)/(n_1 + n_2)}$$

Sometimes we have paired data where two experiments are performed in one subject. The variances with paired data are usually smaller than with unpaired because of the positive correlation between two observations in one subject (those who respond well the first time are more likely to do so the second). This phenomenon translates in a slightly modified calculation of variance parameters.

$$\textbf{SD}_{paired\ sum} = \sqrt{(\textbf{SD}_1^2 + \textbf{SD}_2^2 + 2\ r\ \textbf{SD}_1 . \textbf{SD}_2)}$$

$$\textbf{SD}_{paired\ differrence} = \sqrt{(\textbf{SD}_1^2 + \textbf{SD}_2^2 - 2\ r\ \textbf{SD}_1 . \textbf{SD}_2)}$$

Where r = correlation coefficient, a term that will be explained soon.

Likewise

$$\text{SEM}_{\text{paired sum}} = \sqrt{(SD_1^2 + SD_2^2 + 2\,r\,SD_1.\,SD_2)}\,/n$$

$$\text{SEM}_{\text{paired differrence}} = \sqrt{(SD_1^2 + SD_2^2 - 2\,r\,SD_1.\,SD_2)}\,/n$$

where, again, $n = n_1 = n_2$

Note that SEM does not directly quantify variability in a population. A small SEM can be mainly due to a large sample size rather than tight data.

With small samples the distribution of the means does not exactly follow a Gaussian distribution. But rather a t-distribution, 95% confidence intervals cannot be characterized as the area under the curve between mean ± 2 SEMs but instead the area under curve is substantially wider and is characterized as mean ± t.SEMs where t is close to 2 with large samples but 2.5-3 with samples as small as 5-10. The appropriate t for any sample size is given in the socalled t-table.

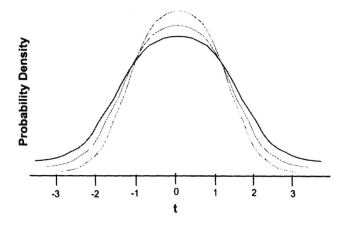

Figure 2. Family of t-distributions: with n=5 the distribution is wide, with n=10 and n=1000 this is increasingly less so.

Figure 3 shows that the t-distribution is wider than the Gaussian distribution with small samples. Mean ± t.SEMs presents the 95 % confidence intervals of the means that many similar samples would produce.

Statistics is frequently used to compare more than 2 samples of data. To estimate whether differences between samples are true or just chance we first assess variances in the data between groups and within groups.

Group	sample size	mean	SD
Group 1	n_1	mean $_1$	SD_1
Group 2	n_2	mean $_2$	SD_2
Group 3	n_3	mean $_3$	SD_3

This procedure may seem somewhat awkward in the beginning but in the next two chapters we will observe that variances, which are no less than estimates of noise in the data, are effectively used to test the probabilities of true differences between, e.g., different pharmaceutical compounds.

Between-group variance:

Sum of squares$_{between}$ = $SS_{between}$ = n_1 (mean$_1$ – overall mean)^2 + n_2(mean$_2$ – overall mean)^2 + n_3 (mean$_3$ – overall mean)^2

Within-group variance:

Sum of squares$_{within}$ = SS_{within} = $(n_1-1) SD_1^2$ + $(n_2-1) SD_2^2$ + $(n_3-1) SD_3^2$

The quotient of the sum of squares between-group / sum of squares within group (after proper adjustment for the sample sizes or degrees of freedom, a term which will be explained later on) is called the big F and determines whether variances between the sample means is larger than expected from the variability within the samples. If so, we reject the null hypothesis of no diffference between the samples. With two samples the square root of big F, which actually is the test statistic of analysis of variance (ANOVA), is equal to the t of the famous t-test, which will further be explained in chapter 2. These 10 or so lines already brought us very close to what is currently considered the heart of statistics, namely ANOVA (analysis of variance).

4. DIFFERENT TYPES OF DATA: PROPORTIONS, PERCENTAGES AND CONTINGENCY TABLES

Instead of continuous data, data may also be of an ordinal character where two or more alternatives are possible, and, generally, the frequencies of occurrence of each of these possibilities are calculated. The simplest and commonest type of ordinal data are the socalled binary data (yes/no etc). Such data are frequently assessed as proportions or percentages, and follow a socalled binomial distribution. If $0.1<$ proportion (p) <0.9 the binomial distribution becomes very close to the normal distribution. If p <0.1, the data will follow a skewed distribution, otherwise called Poisson distribution. Proportional data can be conveniently laid-out as contingency tables.

The simplest contingency table looks like this

	numbers of subjects with side Effect	numbers of subjects without side effect
Test treatment (group$_1$)	a	b
Control treatment (group$_2$)	c	d

The proportion of subjects who had a side effect in group$_1$ (or the risk (**R**) or probability of having an effect)

$$p= a / (a+b) , \text{ in group}_2 \text{ } p= c / (c+d),$$

The quotient of **a / (a+b)** and **c / (c+d)** is called **risk ratio (RR)**

Note that the terms proportion, risk and probability are frequently used in statistical procedures but that they basically mean the same.

Another approach is the **odds** approach **a/b** and **c/d** are odds and their quotient is the **odds ratio(OR)**.
In clinical trials we use ORs as surrogate RRs, because here a/(a+b) is simply nuts.
For example:

	treatment-group	control-group	whole-population
sleepiness	32 a	4 b	4000
no sleepiness	24 c	52 d	52000

We assume that the control group is just a sample from the population but that the ratio b/d is that of the population. So, suppose 4=4000 and 52= 52000, then
$$\frac{a/(a+b)}{c/(c+d)} = \frac{a/b}{c/d} = RR \text{ of the population.}$$

Proportions can also be expressed as percentages:

$$\text{p.100 \%= a / (a+b). (100\%) etc}$$

Just as with continuous data we can calculate SDs and SEMs and 95% confidence intervals of rates (or numbers, or scores) and of proportions or percentages.

$$\text{SD of number n} = \sqrt{n}$$
$$\text{SD of difference between two numbers } n_1 \text{ and } n_2 = n_1\text{-}n_2/\sqrt{(n_1+n_2)}$$
$$\text{SD proportion} = \sqrt{p(1-p)}$$

$$\text{SEM proportion} = \sqrt{p\,(1\text{-}p)\,/\,n}$$

We assume that the distribution of proportions of many samples follows a normal distribution (in this case called the z-distribution) with 95% confidence intervals between

$$p \pm 2\sqrt{p\,/\,(1\text{-}p)\,/\,n}$$

a formula looking very similar to the 95% CI intervals formula for continuous data

$$\text{mean} \pm 2\sqrt{SD^2\,/\,n}$$

Differences and sums of the SDs and SEMs of proportions can be calculated similarly to those of continuous data

$$\text{SEM of differences} = \sqrt{p_1\,/\,(1\text{-}p_1)\,/\,n_1 + p_2\,/\,(1\text{-}p_2)\,/\,n_2}$$

with 95% CI intervals : $p_1 - p_2 \pm 2.\,\text{SEMs}$

More often than with continuous data, proportions of different samples are assessed for their quotient rather than difference or sum. Calculating the 95% CI intervals of it is not simple. The problem is that the quotient-of-many- samples does not have a normal distribution, and is extremely skewed. It can never be less than 0 but can get very high. However, the logarithm of the relative risk is approximately symmetrical. Katz's method takes advantage of this symmetry:

$$\text{95\% CI of log RR} = \log RR \pm 2 \sqrt{\frac{b/a}{a+b} + \frac{d/c}{c+d}}$$

This equation calculates the CIs of the logarithm of the RR. Take the antilogarithm (10^x) to determine the 95% CIs of the RR.

Probability distribution

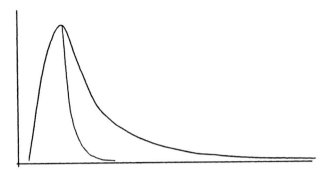

Figure 4. Ratios of proportions unlike continuous data usually do not have a normal but a skewed distribution (values vary from 0 to ∞). Transformation into the logarithms provides approximately symmetric distributions.

Figure 3 shows the distribution of RRs and the distribution of the logarithms of the RRs, and illustrate that the transformation from skewed data into their logarithms is a useful method to obtain an approximately symmetrical distribution, that can be analyzed according to the usual approach of SDs, SEMs and CIs.

5. DIFFERENT TYPES OF DATA: CORRELATION COEFFICIENT

The SD and SEM of paired data includes a term called r as described above. For the calculation of r we have to take into account that paired comparisons, e.g., those of two drugs tested in one subject generally have a different variance from those of comparison of two drugs in two different subjects. This is so, because between subject variability of symptoms is eliminated and because the chance of a subject responding beneficially the first time is more likely to respond beneficially the second time as well. We say there is generally a positive correlation between the response of one subject to two treatments.

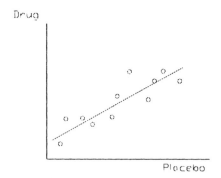

Figure 5. A positive correlation between the
response of one subject to two treatments

Figure 4 gives an example of this phenomenon. X-variables, e.g., blood pressures after the administration of compound 1, y-variables blood pressures after the administration of compound 2 or placebo.

The SDs and SEMs of the paired sums or differences of the x- and y-variables are relevant to estimate variances in the data and are just as those of continuous data needed before any statistical test can be performed. They can be calculated according to:

$$\text{SD}_{\text{paired sum}} = \sqrt{(\text{SD}_1^2 + \text{SD}_2^2 + 2\, r\, \text{SD}_1.\, \text{SD}_2)}$$

$$\text{SD}_{\text{paired differrence}} = \sqrt{(\text{SD}_1^2 + \text{SD}_2^2 - 2\, r\, \text{SD}_1.\, \text{SD}_2)}$$

Where r = correlation coefficient, a term that will be explained soon.

Likewise

$$\text{SEM}_{\text{paired sum}} = \sqrt{(\text{SD}_1^2 + \text{SD}_2^2 + 2\, r\, \text{SD}_1.\, \text{SD}_2)} \, /n$$

$$\text{SEM}_{\text{paired differrence}} = \sqrt{(\text{SD}_1^2 + \text{SD}_2^2 - 2\, r\, \text{SD}_1.\, \text{SD}_2)} \, /n$$

where $n = n_1 = n_2$

and that

$$r = \frac{\Sigma\,(x - \bar{x})\,(y - \bar{y})}{\sqrt{\Sigma\,(x - \bar{x})^2\,\,(y - \bar{y})^2}}$$

r is between −1 and +1, and with unpaired data r=0 and the SD and SEM formulas reduce accordingly (as described above). The figure also shows a line, called the regression line, which presents the best-fit summary of the data, and is the calculated method that minimizes the squares of the distances from the line.

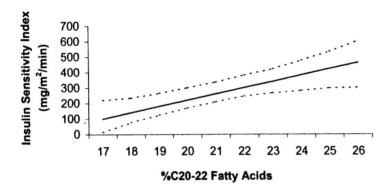

*Figure 6. Example of a linear regression line of 2 paired variables
(x- and y-values), the regression line provides the best fit line.
The dotted curves are 95% CIs that are curved, although we do
not allow for a nonlinear relationship between x and y variables.*

The 95% CIs of a regression line can be calculated and is drawn as area between the dotted lines in Figure 5. It is remarkable that the borders of the straight regression line are curved although we do not allow for a nonlinear relationship between the x-axis and y-axis variables. More details on regression analysis will be given in chapters 2 and 3.

In the above few lines we described continuous normally distributed or t-distributed data, and rates and their proportions or percentages. We did not yet address data ordered as ranks. This is a special method to transform skewed data into a approximately normal distribution, and is in that sense comparable with logarithmic transformation of relative risks (RRs). In chapter 3 the tests involving this method will be explained.

6. STRATIFICATION ISSUES

When published, a randomized parallel-group drug trial essentially includes a table listing all of the factors, otherwise called baseline characteristics, known possibly to influence outcome. E.g., in case of heart disease these will probably include apart from age and gender, the prevalence in each group of diabetes, hypertension, cholesterol levels, smoking history. If such factors are similar in the two groups, then we can go on to attribute any difference in outcome to the effect of test-treatment over reference –treatment. If not, we have a problem. Attempts are made to retrieve the situation by multivariate analysis allocating part of the differences in outcome to the differences in the groups, but there is always an air of uncertainty about the validity of the overall conclusions in such a trial. This issue is discussed and methods are explained in chapter 8. Here we discuss ways to avoid this problem. Ways to do so, are stratification of the analysis and minimization of imbalance between treatment groups, which are both techniques not well-known. Stratification of the analysis means that relatively homogeneous subgroups are analyzed separately. The limitation of this approach is that it can not account for more than two, maybe three, variables and that thus major covariates may be missed. Minimization can manage many more factors. The investigators first classify patients according to the factors they would like to see equally presented in the two groups, then randomly assign treatment so that predetermined approximately fixed proportions of patients from each stratum receive each treatment. With this method the group allocation does not rely solely on chance but is designed to reduce any difference in the distribution of unsuspected contributing determinants of outcome so that any treatment difference can now be attributed to the treatment comparison itself. A good example of this method can be found in a study by Kallis et al. [1] The authors stratified in a study of aspirin versus placebo before coronary artery surgery the groups according to age, gender, left ventricular function, and number of coronary arteries affected. Any other prognostic factors other than treatment can be chosen. If the treatments are given in a double-blind fashion, minimization influences the composition of the two groups but does not influence the chance of one group entering in a particular treatment arm rather than the other.

There is an additional argument in favor of stratification/ minimization that counts even if the risk of significant asymmetries in the treatment groups is small. Some prognostic factors have a particularly large effect on the outcome of a trial. Even small and statistically unsignificant imbalances in the treatment groups may then bias the results. E.g., in a study of two treatment modalities for pneumonia[2] including 54 patients, 10 patients took prior antibiotic in the treatment group and 5 did in the control group. Even though the difference between 5/27 and 10/27 is not statistically significant, the validity of this trial was being challenged, and the results were eventually not accepted.

7. RANDOMIZED VERSUS HISTORICAL CONTROLS

A randomized clinical trial is frequently used in drug research. However, there is considerable opposition to the use of this design. One major concern is the ethical problem of allowing a random event to determine a patient's treatment. Freirich[3] argued that a comparative trial which shows major differences between two treatments is a bad trial because half of the patients have received an inferior treatment. On the other hand in a prospective trial randomly assigning treatments avoids many potential biases. Of more concern is the trial in which a new treatment is compared to an old treatment when there is information about the efficacy of the old treatment through historical data. In this situation use of the historical data for comparisons with data from the new treatment will shorten the length of the study because all patients can be assigned to the new treatment. The current availibility of multivariate statistical procedures which can adjust the comparison of two treatments for differing presence of other prognostic factors in the two treatment arms, has made the use of historical controls more appealing. This has made randomization less necessary as a mechanism for ensuring comparability of the treatment arms. The weak point in this approach is the absolute faith one has to place in the multivariate model. Also, some confounding variables e.g., time effects, simply can not be adjusted, and remain unknown. Despite the ethical argument in favor of historical controls we must therefore emphasize the potentially misleading aspects of trials using historical controls.

8. FACTORIAL DESIGNS

The majority of drug trials are designed to answer a single question. However, in practice many diseases require a combination of more than one treatment modalities. E.g., beta-blockers are effective for stable angina pectoris but beta-blockers plus calcium channel blockers or beta-blockers plus calcium channel blockers plus nitrates are better (table 1). Not addressing more than one treatment modality in a trial is an unnecessary restriction on the design of the trial because the assessment of two or more modalities in on a trial pose no major mathematical problems.

Table 1.The factorial design for angina pectoris patients treated with calcium channel blockers with or without beta-blockers

	Calcium channel blocker	no calcium channel blocker
Beta-blocker	regimen I	regimen II
No beta-blocker	regimen III	regimen I

We will not describe the analytical details of such a design but researchers should not be reluctant to consider designs of such types. This is particularly so, when the recruitment of large samples causes difficulties.

9. REFERENCES

1. Kallis F et al. Aspirin versus placebo before coronary artery surgery. Eur J
   Cardiovasc Surg 1994; 8: 404-10.
2. Graham WG, Bradley DA. Efficacy of chest physiotherapy and intermittent
   positive-pressure breathing in the resolution of pneumonia.
   N Engl J Med 1978; 299: 624-7.
3. Freirich F. Ethical problem of allowing a random event to determine a patient's
   treatment. In: Controversies in clinical trials. Saunders, Philadelphia, 1983, p 5.

CHAPTER 2

THE ANALYSIS OF EFFICACY DATA OF DRUG TRIALS

1. OVERVIEW

Typical efficacy endpoints have their associated statistical techniques. For example, values of continuous measurements (e.g., blood pressure) require the following statistical techniques:
a. if measurements are normally distributed: t-tests and associated confidence intervals to compare two mean values; analysis of variance (ANOVA) to compare three or more.
b. If measurements have a non-normal distribution: Wilcoxon rank tests with confidence intervals for medians.

Comparing proportions of responders or proportions of survivors or patients with no events involves binomial rather than normal distributions and requires a completely different approach. It requires a chi-square test, or a more complex technique otherwise closely related to the simple chi-square test, e.g., Mantel Haenszl summary chi-square test, logrank test, Cox proportional hazard test etc. Although in clinical trials particularly phase III-IV trials proportions of responders and proportion of survivors is increasingly an efficacy endpoint, in many other trials proportions are used mainly for the purpose of assessing safety endpoints, while continous measurements are used for assessing the main endpoints, mostly efficacy endpoints. We will therefore focus on statistically testing continuous measurements in this chapter and will deal with different aspects of statistically testing proportions in the next chapter.
Statistical tests all have in common that they try to estimate the probability that a difference in the data is true rather than due to chance. Usually statistical tests make use of a socalled **test statistic**

Chi-square	for the chi-square test
t	for the t-test
Q	for nonparametric comparisons
Q^1	for nonparametric comparisons
q	for Neuman-Keuls test
q^1	for Dunnett test
F	for analysis of variance
Rs	for Spearman rank correlation test

These test statistics can adopt different sizes. In the appendix of this book we present tables for t-, chi-square- and F- , Mann-Whitney-, and Wilcoxon-rank-sum-tests, but additional tables are published in most textbooks of statistics (see References). Such tables show us the larger the size of the test statistic, the more likely it is that the null hypothesis of no difference from zero or no difference between two samples is untrue, and that there is thus a true difference or true effect in the data. Most tests also have in common that they are better sensitive or powerful to demonstrate such a true difference as the samples tested are large. So, the test statistic in most tables is adjusted for sample sizes. We say that the sample size determines the degrees of freedom, a term closely related to the sample size.

2. THE PRINCIPLE OF TESTING STATISTICAL SIGNIFICANCE,

The human brain excels in making hypotheses but hypotheses may be untrue. When you were a child you thought that only girls could become doctor because your family doctor was a female. Later on, this hypothesis proved to be untrue. Hypotheses must be assessed with hard data. Statistical analyses of hard data starts with assumptions:

1. our study is representative for the entire population (if we repeat the trial, difference will be negligible.
2. All similar trials will have the same SD or SEM.

Because biological processes *full* of variations, statistics gives no certainties only chances. What chances? Chances that hypotheses are true/untrue. What hypotheses?: e.g.

1. our mean effect is not different from a 0 effect.
2. It is really different from a 0 effect.
3. It is worse than a 0 effect.

Statistics is about estimating such chances / testing such hypotheses. Please note that trials often calculate differences between a test treatment and a control treatment and, subsequently, test whether this difference is larger than 0. Thus, a simple way to reduce a study of two groups of data and thus two means to a single mean and single distribution of data, is to take the difference between the two and compare it with 0.

In the past chapter we explained that the data of a trial can be described in the form of a normal distribution graph with SEMs on the x-axis, and that this method is adequate to test various statistical hypotheses. We will now focus on a very important hypothesis, the null-hypothesis. What it literally means is: no difference from a 0 effect. We will try and make a graph of this null-hypothesis.

What does it look in graph? H1 in Figure 1 is a graph based on the data of our trial with SEMs distant from mean on the x-axis (z-axis). H0 is the same graph with a mean value of 0 (mean ± SEM= 0 ± 1). Now we make a giant leap from our data to

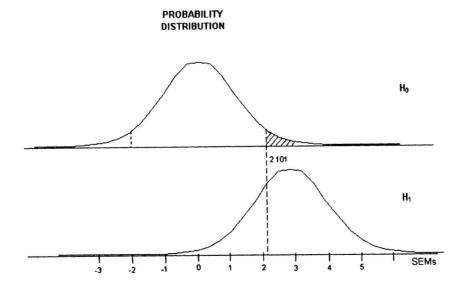

Figure 1. Null-hypothesis (H₀) and alternative hypothesis H₁ of an example of experimental data with sample size (n) = 20 and mean = 2.9 SEMs, and a t-distributed frequency distribution.

the entire population, and we can do so, because our data are representative for the entire population. H1 is also the summary of the means of many trials similar to ours (if we repeat, differences will be small, and summary will look alike). H0 is also the summary of the means of many trials similar to ours but with an overall effect of 0. Now our mean effect is not 0 but 2.9. Yet it could be an outlier of many studies with an overall effect of 0. So, we should think from now on of H0 as the distribution of the means of many trials with overall effect of 0. If H0 is true, then the mean of our study is part of H0. We can not prove anything, but we can calculate the chance/probability of this possibility.

A mean value of 2.9 is far distant from 0. Suppose it belangs to H0. Only 5% of the H0 trials have their means >2.1 SEMs distant from 0, because AUC>2.1 distant from 0 is 5% of total AUC. Thus, the chance that our mean belongs to H0 is <5%. This is a small chance, and we reject this chance and conclude there is <5% chance to find this result. We, thus, reject the H0 of no difference from 0 at P<0.05. The AUC right from 2.101 is called alpha= area of rejection of H0. Our result of 2.9 is far from 2.101. The probability of finding such a result may be a lot smaller than 5%. Table 1 shows the t-table that can tell us exactly how small this chance truly is.

Table 1. t-table

df	Two-tailed P-value			
	0.10	0.05	0.01	0.001
1	6.314	12.706	63.656	636.58
2	2.920	4.303	9.925	31.600
3	2.353	3.182	5.841	12.924
4	2.132	2.776	4.604	8.610
5	2.015	2.571	4.032	6.869
6	1.943	2.447	3.707	5.959
7	1.895	2.365	3.499	5.408
8	1.860	2.306	3.355	5.041
9	1.833	2.262	3.250	4.781
10	1.812	2.228	3.169	4.587
11	1.796	2.201	3.106	4.437
12	1.782	2.179	3.055	4.318
13	1.771	2.160	3.012	4.221
14	1.761	2.145	2.977	4.140
15	1.753	2.131	2.947	4.073
16	1.746	2.120	2.921	4.015
17	1.740	2.110	2.898	3.965
18	1.734	2.101	2.878	3.922
19	1.729	2.093	2.861	3.883
20	1.725	2.086	2.845	3.850
21	1.721	2.080	2.831	3.819
22	1.717	2.074	2.819	3.792
23	1.714	2.069	2.807	3.768
24	1.711	2.064	2.797	3.745
25	1.708	2.060	2.787	3.725
26	1.706	2.056	2.779	3.707
27	1.703	2.052	2.771	3.689
28	1.701	2.048	2.763	3.674
29	1.699	2.045	2.756	3.660
30	1.697	2.042	2.750	3.646
40	1.684	2.021	2.704	3.551
50	1.676	2.009	2.678	3.496
100	1.660	1.984	2.626	3.390
200	1.653	1.972	2.601	3.340
5000	1.645	1.960	2.577	3.293

The 4 right-hand columns are trial results expressed in SEM-units distant from 0 (=**also t-values**). The upper row are the AUC-values right from trial results. The left-hand column presents adjustment for numbers of patients (degrees of freedom (dfs), in our example two samples of 10 gives 20-2:= 18 dfs).

AUC right from 2.9 means→ right from 2.878 means→ this AUC<0.01. And so we conclude that our probability not <0.05 but even<0.01.Note: the t-distribution is just an adjustment of the normal distribution, but a bit wider for small samples. With large samples it is identical to the normal distribution. For proportional data always the normal distribution is applied.

3. UNPAIRED T-TEST

So far, we asessed a single mean versus 0, now we assess two means versus each other. For example, a parallel-group study of two groups tests the effect of two beta-blockers on cardiac output.

	Mean ± SD			$SEM^2=SD^2/n$
group 1 (n=10)	5.9	± 2.4	liter/min	5.76/10
group 2 (n=10)	4.5	± 1.7	liter/min	2.89/10

Calculate: mean - mean = 1.4

Then calculate pooled SEM= $\sqrt{(SEM_1^2 + SEM_2^2)}$ = $1.4 \pm \sqrt{0.433}$ = 1.4 ± 0.658

Note: for SEM of difference: take the square root of the sums of squares of separate SEMs and so reduce analysis of two eans and two SEMS to one of a single one.

$$\text{The size of } t = \frac{\text{mean}_1 - \text{mean}_2}{\text{pooled SEM}} = 1.4 / 0.658 = 2.127$$

So, significance of difference between two unpaired samples of continuous data is best assessed by the formula

$$\text{Difference: } \textbf{mean}_1 - \textbf{mean}_2 \pm \sqrt{(\textbf{SEM}_1^2 + \textbf{SEM}_2^2)}$$

This formula presents again a t-distribution with a new mean and a new SEM. The wider this new mean is distant from zero and the smaller its SEM is, the more likely we are able to demonstrate a true effect or true difference from no effect. The size of the test statistic is actually calculated as mean/SEM. With n=20 the t-table shows that a t of 2.101 provides a chance of 5% that the null hypothesis of no effect can be rejected.

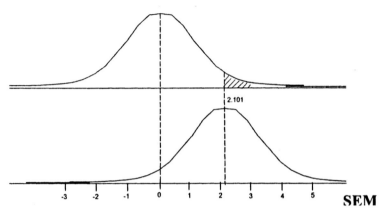

Figure 2. Two t- distributions with n=20: lower curve H1 or actual SEM-distribution of the data, upper curve H0 or null hypothesis of the study.

The lower graph (H1 of Figure 2) is the probability distribution of this t-distribution. H0 (the upper graph) is an identical distribution with mean= 0 instead of mean = $mean_1$-$mean_2$ and with SEM identical to the SEM of H1, and is taken as the null hypothesis in this particular approach. With n=20 (18 dfs)we can accept that 95% of all t-distributions with no significant treatment difference from zero must have their means between –2.101 and +2.101 SEMs from zero. The chance of finding a mean value of + 2.101 SEMs or more is 5% or less (we say α=0.05, where α is the chance of erroneously rejecting the null hypothesis of no effect). This means that we can reject the null hypothesis of no difference at a probability (P) =0.05. We have 5% chance of coming to this result, if there were no difference between the two samples. We, therefore, conclude that there is a true difference between the effects of the two compounds on cardiac output.

Also the F- and chi-square test reject, similarly to the t-test, reject the null hypothesis of no treatment effect if the value of the test statistic is bigger than 95% of the values that would occur if the treatment had no effect. At this point we should emphasize that when the test statistic is not big enough to reject the null hypothesis of no treatment effect, investigators often report no statistically significant difference and discuss their results in terms of documented proof that the treatment had no effect. All they really did, was, fail to demonstrate that it did have an effect. The distinction between positively demonstrating that a treatment had no effect and failing to demonstrate that it does have an effect, is subtle but very important, especially with respect to the small numbers of subjects usually enrolled in a trial. A study of treatments that involves only a few subjects and then fails to reject the null hypothesis of no treatment effect, may arrive at that conclusion because the statistical procedure lacked power to detect the effect because of a too small sample size, even though the treatment did have an effect. We will address this problem in more detail in chapter 5.

4. NULL HYPOTHESIS TESTING OF 3 OR MORE UNPAIRED SAMPLES

If more than two samples are compared, things soon get really complicated, and the unpaired t-test can no longer be applied. Usually, statistical software, e.g., SAS or SPSS Statistical Software, will be used to produce F- or P-values, but the table 2 gives a brief summary of the principles of multiple groups analysis of variance (ANOVA) applied for this purpose.

Table 2. Multiple groups ANOVA

Unpaired ANOVA 3 groups

                        Total variation
                    | |
        Between group variation   within group variation

In ANOVA:

Variations expressed as sums of squares (SS) and can be added up to obtain total variation. Assess whether between-group variation is large compared to within-.

Group	n patients	mean	SD
1	-	-	-
2	-	-	-
3	-	-	-

Grand mean = (mean 1 + 2 +3)/3

$SS_{between\ groups} = n_1\ (\ mean_1 - grand\ mean)^2 + n_2\ (\ mean_2 - grand\ mean)^2 + ...$

$SS_{within\ groups} = (n_1-1)(SD_1^2) + (n_2-1)\ SD_2^2 + ...$

$$F = \frac{SS_{between\ groups}\ /\ dfs}{SS_{within\ groups}\ /\ dfs} = MS_{between}\ /\ MS_{within}$$

F-table gives P-value

Effect of 3 compounds on Hb

Group	n patients	mean	SD
1	16	8.7125	0.8445
2	10	10.6300	1.2841
3	15	12.3000	0.9419

Grand mean = (mean 1 + 2 +3)/3 = 10.4926

$SS_{between\ groups} = 16\ (8.7125-10.4926)^2 + 10(10.6300 - 10.4926)^2 ....$

$SS_{within\ groups} = 15 \times 0.8445^2 + 10 \times 1.2841^2 + ...$

$F = 49.9$ and so $P < 0.001$

Note: In case 2 groups: ANOVA= unpaired T-test $(F=T^2)$. Dfs means degrees of freedom, and equals $n_1 + n_2 + n_3 - 3$ for SS_{within}, and 3-1=2 for $SS_{between}$.

5. THREE METHODS TO TEST STATISTICALLY A PAIRED SAMPLE

Table 3 gives an example of a placebo-controlled clinical trial to test efficacy of sleeping drug.

Table 3. Example of a placebo-controlled clinical trial to test efficacy of sleeping drug

	hours of sleep				
patient	drug	placebo	difference	mean	SS
1	6.1	5.2	0.9	5.7	0.53
2	7.0	7.9	−0.9	7.5	
3	8.2	3.9	4.3		
4	7.6	4.7	2.9		
5	6.5	5.3	1.2		
6	7.8	5.4	3.0		
7	6.9	4.2	2.7		
8	6.7	6.1	0.6		
9	7.4	3.8	3.6		
10	5.8	6.3	−0.5		
Mean	7.06	5.28	1.78		
SD	0.76	1.26	1.77		
grand mean	6.17				

FIRST METHOD

First method is simply calculating the SD of the mean difference $\overline{d}$ by looking at the row of differences (d´s) and using the standard formula for variance between data

$$\text{SD paired differences} = \sqrt{[\,\Sigma\,(d - \overline{d}\,)^2 / (n\text{-}1)]} = 1.79 \ .$$

Next we find SEM of the mean difference by taking SD/$\sqrt{n}$=0.56
Mean difference ± SEM= 1.78 ± 0.56
Similarly to the above unpaired t-test we now can test the null hypothesis of no difference by calculating

Mean difference

$t = \dfrac{\text{Mean difference}}{\text{SEM}}$ $= 1.78 / 0.56 = 3.18$ with a sample of 10 (degrees of freedom = 10-1).

The t-table shows that $P<0.02$. We have <2% chance to find this result if there were no difference, and accept that this is sufficient to assume that there is a true difference.

SECOND METHOD

Instead of taking the row of differences we can take the other two rows and use the formula as described in chapter 1 for calculating the SD of the paired differences=$SD_{\text{paired differrence}}$

$$= \sqrt{(SD_1{}^2 + SD_2{}^2 - 2\, r\, SD_1.\, SD_2)}$$
$$= \sqrt{(0.76^2 + 1.26^2 - 2 \times r \times 0.76 \times 1.26)}$$

As r can be calculated to be +0.26, we can now conclude that

$SD_{\text{paired differrence}} = 1.79$

The rest of the calculations is as above.

THIRD METHOD

The third method is ANOVA. We have to calculate SS (sum of squares) e.g., for subject 1:

$SS_{\text{wit subj 1}} = (6.1\text{-}5.7)^2 + (5.2\text{-}5.7)^2 = 0.53$

grand mean $(7.06+5.28)/\,2 = 6.17$

$SS_{\text{wit subj}} = SS_{\text{wit subj 1}} + SS_{\text{wit subj 2}} + SS_{\text{wit subj 3}} + \ldots.$

$SS_{\text{bet subj}} = 2[(5.7\text{-}6.17)^2 + (7.45\text{-}6.17)^2 + (\ldots$ Note: 2 is number of treatments.

$SS_{\text{treat}} = 10[\ (7.06\text{-}6.17)^2 + (5.28\text{-}6.17)^2]$ Note: 10 is the number of patients to compute each mean.

$SS_{\text{res}} = SS_{\text{wit subj}} - SS_{\text{treat}}$

Table 4. ANOVA table of these data

Source of variation	Sum of Squares (SS)	degrees of freedom (d.f.)	mean square MS=SS/d.f.)	$F = \dfrac{\text{MS treatment}}{\text{MS residual}}$
between subjects		2 (m)		
within subjects		10 (n x (m-1))		
treatments		1 (m-1)		F= 7.28, p<0.02
residual		9 (n-1)		
total		22		

Note m is number of treatments, n is number of patients. The ANOVA is valid not only for two repeated measures but also for m repeated measures. For 2 repeated measures it is actually equal to the paired t-test.

Similarly, for unpaired samples, with two samples the one way ANOVA already briefly mentioned in chapter 1 is equal to the unpaired t-test, but one-way ANOVA can also be used for m unpaired samples.

The above data can also be presented in the form of a linear regression graph.

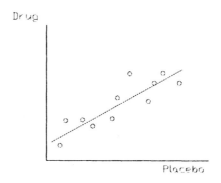

Figure 3. Paired data layed out in the form of linear regression.

Paired data can also be layed out in the form of linear regression

    y=a+bx   (effect drug) = a+ b (effect placebo)

which can be assessed in the form of ANOVA:

$$F = r^2 = \frac{\text{regression sum of squares}}{\text{total sum of squares}} = \frac{(\Sigma(x - \overline{x})(y - \overline{y}))^2}{\Sigma(x - \overline{x})^2 \cdot \Sigma(y - \overline{y})^2} = \frac{SP^2 \; x \cdot y \text{ -values}}{SS \; x \text{ -values} \cdot SS \; y \text{ -values}}$$

SS regression= SP^2 x . y -values / SS x -values
SS total = SS y
SS regression / SS total = r^2

Table 5. ANOVA table for the linear regression between paired samples

Source of variation	Sum of Squares (SS)	degrees of freedom (d.f.)	mean square MS=SS/d.f.	MS regression F = ─────── MS total
regression between samples	1.017	1	1.017	0.58, P>0.05
residual	14.027	8	1.753	
total	15.044	9		

The ANOVA table (table 5) gives an alternative interpretation of the correlation coefficient; the square of the correlation coefficient, r, equals the regression sum of squares divided by the total sum of squares ($0.26^2 = 0.0676 = 1.017/15.044$) and, thus, is the proportion of the total variation that has been explained by the regression. We can say that the variances in the drug data are only for 6.76% determined by the variances in the placebo data, and that they are for 93.24% independent of the placebo data. With strong positive correlations ,e.g., close to +1 the formula for SD and thus SEM reduces to a very small size (because [$SD_1^2 + SD_2^2 - 2 \, r \, SD_1. \, SD_2$] will be close to zero), and the paired t-test produces huge sizes of t and thus huge sensitivity of testing. The above approach cannot be used for estimating significance of differences between two paired samples. And the method in the presented form is not very relevant. It starts, however, to be relevant, if we we are interested in the dependency of a particular outcome variable upon several factors. E.g., the effect of drug is better than placebo but this effect still gets better with increased age. This concept can be represented by a multiple regression equation

$$y = a + b_1 x_1 + b_2 x_2$$

which in this example is

drug response= a + b_1 . (placebo response) + b_2 . (age)

Although it is no longer easy to visualize the regression, the principles involved are the same as with linear regression. In chapter 8 this subject will be dealt with more explicitly.

6. NULL-HYPOTHESIS TESTING OF 3 OR MORE PAIRED SAMPLES

If more than two paired samples are compared, things soon get really complicated, and the paired t-test can no longer be applied. Usually, statistical software (SAS, SPSS) will be used to produce F- and P-values, but the table 6 gives a brief summary of the principles of ANOVA for multiple paired observations, used for this purpose.

Table 6. Repeated measurements ANOVA

Paired ANOVA 3 treatments in single group

$$\text{Total variation}$$

Between subj variation   Within-subj variation

Between treatment variation   Residual variation
(random)

Variations expressed as sums of squares (SS) and can be added up
Assess whether between tr. variation is large compared to resid.

Subj	treatment 1	treatment 2	treatment 3	SD^2
1	-	-	-	-
2	-	-	-	-
3	-	-	-	-
4	-	-	-	-
Treatment mean	-	-		

Grand mean = (treatment mean 1 + 2 + 3)/ 3= .....

$SS_{\text{within subj}}= SD_1^2+SD_2^2+SD_3^2$

$SS_{\text{treatment}} = (\text{treatment mean 1} - \text{grand mean})^2 + (\text{treatment mean 2} - \text{grand mean})^2 + ...$

$SS_{\text{residual}} = SS_{\text{within subj}} - SS_{\text{treatm}}$

$$F= \frac{SS_{\text{treatment}} / \text{dfs}}{SS_{\text{residual}} / \text{dfs}}$$

F table gives P-value.

Effect of 3 treatments on vascular resistance (RR:CO).

Person	treatment 1	treatment 2	treatment 3	SD^2
1	22.2	5.4	10.6	147.95
2	17.0	6.3	6.2	77.05
3	14.1	8.5	9.3	18.35
4	17.0	10.7	12.3	21.4
Treatment mean	17.58	7.73	9.60	

Grand mean = 11.63

$SS_{within\ subj}= 147.95 + 77.05 +....$
$SS_{treatment} = (17.58 - 11.63)^2 + (7.73 - 11.63)^2 +....$
$SS_{residual} = SS_{within\ subj} - SS_{treatm}$

$F= 14.31$ and so $P<0.01$

Note: in case of 2 treatments: repeated measurements-ANOVA paired T-test ($F=T^2$), dfs= degrees of freedom equals 3-1=2 for SStreatment, and 4-1=3 for SSresidual.

7. PAIRED DATA WITH A NEGATIVE CORRELATION

Many crossover and parallel-group studies include an element of self-controlling. E.g., observations before, during, and after treatment are frequently used as the main control on experimental variation. Such repeated measures will generally have a positive correlation: those who respond well during the first observation are more likely to do so in the second. This is, however, not necessarily so. When drugs of completely different classes are compared, patients may fall apart into different populations: those who respond better to one and those who respond better to the other drug. For example, patients with angina pectoris, hypertension, arrhythmias, chronic obstructive pulmonary disease, unresponsive to one class of drugs, may respond very well to a different class of drugs. This situation gives rise to a negative correlation in a paired comparison. Other examples of negative correlations between paired observations include the following. A negative correlation between subsequent observations in one subject may occur because fast-responders are more likely to stop responding earlier. A negative correlation may exist in the patient characteristics of a trial, e.g., between age and vital lung capacity, and in outcome variables of a trial, e.g., between severity of heart attack and ejection fraction. Negative correlations in a paired comparison reduce the sensitivity not only of studies testing significance but also of studies testing equivalence.

I: STUDIES TESTING SIGNIFICANCE

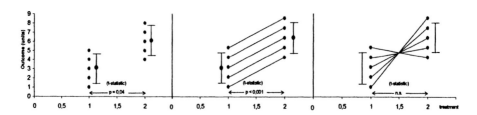

Figure 4. Hypothesized examples of three studies: left graph parallel-group study of 10 patients, middle and right graphs self-controlled studies of 5 patients each tested twice.

Figure 4 gives a hypothesized example of three studies: the left graph shows a parallel-group study of 10 patients, the middle and right graph show self-controlled studies of 5 patients each tested twice. T-statistics is employed according to the formula

$$t \ = \ \frac{d}{SE}$$

Where d is the mean difference between the two sets of data (6-3=3) and the standard error (SE) of this difference is calculated for the left graph data according to

$$\sqrt{\frac{SD_1^2}{n_1} + \frac{SD_2^2}{n_2}} = 0.99$$

SD_1 and SD_2 are standard deviations and n_1 and n_2 are numbers of observations in each of the groups. We assume that $n_1 = n_2 = n$.

$$t = 3 / 0.99 = 3.0$$

With 10 observations we can reject the null-hypothesis at p = 0.04.
With a positively paired comparison (middle graph) we have even more sensitivity. SE is calculated slightly different

$$SE = \frac{\sqrt{\Sigma (d - \overline{d})^2 / (n -1)}}{\sqrt{n}} = 0$$

where d is the observed change in each individual and $\overline{d}$ is its mean.

$$t = \overline{d} / SE = 3/0 = \infty$$

with n=5 we can reject the null-hypothesis at p<0.001.

The right graph gives the negative correlation situation. SE calculated similarly to the middle graph data is 1.58, which means that

$$t = 3 / 1.58 = 1.89$$

The null-hypothesis of no difference cannot be rejected. Differences are not significant (n.s.).

When more than 2 treatments are given to one sample of patients t-statistics is not appropriate and should be replaced by analysis of variance.

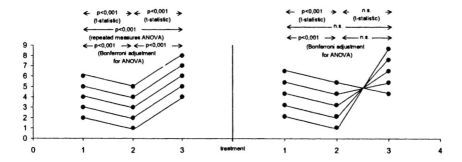

Figure 5. Hypothesized example of two studies where 5 patients are tested three times. Due to negative correlation between treatment 2 and 3 in the right study, the statistical significance test is negative unlike the left graph study, despite the identical mean results.

Figure 5 gives a hypothesized example of two studies where 5 patients are tested three times. In the left graph the correlation between treatment responses is positive, whereas in the right graph the correlation between treatment no.3 and no.2 is strong negative rather than positive. For the left graph data repeated measures ANOVA is performed.

The sum of squares (SS) of the different treatments is calculated according to

Patient	treatment 1	treatment 2	treatment 3	Mean	SS
1	6	5	8	6.3	4.67
2	5	4	7	5.3	4.67
3	4	3	6	4.3	4.67
4	3	2	5	3.3	4.67
5	2	1	4	2.3	4.67
Treatment mean	4	3	6		

Grand mean 4.3 $SS_{within\ subjects}$ 23.3

$SS_{treatments} = 5 \, [(4\text{-}4.3)^2+(3\text{-}4.3)^2+(6\text{-}4.3)^2] = 23.35$

$SS_{residual} = SS_{within\ subjects} - SS_{treatments} = 0$

Table 7. ANOVA table of the data

Source of variation	SS	DF	MS
Within subjects	23.35	10	
Treatments	23.35	2	11.68
Residual	0	8	0

$$F = \frac{MS_{treatments}}{MS_{residual}} = \infty \qquad p<0.001$$

This analysis permits concluding that at least one of the treatments produces a change. To isolate which one, we need to use a multiple-comparisons proce dure, e.g., the modified Bonferroni t-test for ANOVA where

"$SE=\Sigma(d -\overline{d})^{2} / (n-1)$" is replaced with "$MS_{residual}$". So, to compare, e.g., treatment no. 2 with treatment no. 3

$$t = \frac{6-3}{\sqrt{2(MS_{residual})/n}} = \infty \qquad p<0.001$$

Of the right graph a similar analysis is performed.

Patients	treatment 1	treatment 2	treatment 3	Mean	SS
1	6	5	4	5.0	1.0
2	5	4	5	4.7	0.67
3	4	3	6	4.3	4.67
4	3	2	7	4.0	14.0
5	2	1	8	3.7	28.49
Treatment mean	4	3	6		

Grand mean 4.3 $SS_{within\ subjects}$ 48.83

$SS_{treatments} = 5 [(4-4.3)^{2}+(3-4.3)^{2}+(6-4.3)^{2}] = 23.35$
$SS_{residual} = SS_{within\ subjects} - SS_{treatments} = 48.83 - 23.35 = 24.48$

Table 8. ANOVA table of the data

Source of variation	SS	DF	MS
Within subjects	48.83	10	
Treatments	23.35	2	11.7
Residual	24.48	8	3.1

$$F = \frac{MS_{treatments}}{MS_{residual}} = 3.77 \qquad p = 0.20$$

This analysis does not permit concluding that one of the treatments produces a change (table 8). The Bonferroni adjustment of treatments no. 2 and no. 3 of course, does not either ($p = 0.24$ and $p = 0.34$).

In conclusion, with negative correlations between treatment responses statistical methods including paired t-statistics, repeated measures ANOVA, and Bonferroni adjustments for ANOVA lack sensitivity to demonstrate significant treatment effects. The question why this is so, is not difficult to recognize. With t-statistics and a negative correlation between-patient-variation is almost doubled by taking paired differences. With ANOVA things are similar.

$SS_{within subjects}$ are twice the size of the positive correlation situation while $SS_{treatments}$ are not different. It follows that the positive correlation situation provides a lot more sensitivity to test than the negative correlation situation.

II. STUDIES TESTING EQUIVALENCE

In an equivalence trial the conventional significance test has little relevance: failure to detect a difference does not imply equivalence, and a difference which is detected may not have any clinical relevance and, thus, may not correspond to practical equivalence. In such trials the range of equivalence is usually predefined as an interval from $-D$ to $+D$ distant from a difference of 0. D is often set equal to a difference of undisputed clinical importance, and hence may be above the minimum of clinical interest by a factor two or three. The bioequivalence study design essentially tests both equivalence and superiority/inferiority. Let us assume that in an equivalence trial of vasodilators for Raynaud's phenomenon 10 patients are treated with vasodilator 1 for one week and for a separate period of one week with vasodilator 2. The data below show the numbers of Raynaud attacks per week (table 9).

Table 9. Correlation levels and their influence on sensitivity of statistical tests

	ρ = -1			ρ = 0			ρ =+1	
	vasodilator			vasodilator			vasodilator	
one	two	paired differences	one	two	paired differences	one	two	paired differences
45	10	35	45	40	5	10	10	0
40	15	25	40	35	5	20	15	5
40	15	25	40	35	5	25	15	10
35	20	15	35	30	5	25	20	5
30	25	5	30	25	5	30	25	5
30	25	5	30	10	20	30	25	5
25	30	-5	25	15	10	35	30	5
25	35	-10	25	15	10	40	35	5
20	35	-15	20	20	0	40	35	5
10	40	-30	10	25	-15	40	40	5

♦ means								
30	25	5	30	25	5	30	25	5
♦ SEMs								
3.16	3.16	6.46	3.16	3.16	2.78	3.16	3.16	0.76
♦ t								
0.8			1.8			6.3		
♦ 95% CIs								
± 14.5			±6.3			± 1.7		

SEM=standard error of the mean;
t means level of t according to t-test for paired differences;
CI means confidence interval calculated according to critical t value of t
-distribution for 10-
1 pairs = 9 degrees of freedom (critical t =2.26, 95% CI= 2.26 x SEM);
ρ= correlation coefficient (the Greek letter is often used instead of r if we mean total population instead of our sample).

Although samples have identical means and SEMs (25 ± 3.16 x-axis, 30 ± 3.16 y-axis) their correlation coefficients range from −1 to +1. The null hypothesis of no equivalence is rejected when the 95% CIs are entirely within the prespecified range of equivalence, in our case defined as between −10 and +10.
In the left trial 95% CIs are between −9.5 and + 19.5, and thus the null hypothesis of no equivalence cannot be rejected. In the middle trial 95% CI are between -1.3 and 11.3, while in the right trial 95% CI are between -3.3 and 6.7 . This means that the last trial has a positive outcome:equivalence is demonstrated, the null hypothesis of no equivalence can be rejected. The negative correlation trial and the zero correlation trial despite a small mean difference between the two treatments, are not sensitive to reject the null hypothesis, and this is obviously so because of the wide confidence intervals associated with negative and zero correlations.

8. RANK TESTING

Non-parametric tests are an alternative for ANOVA or t-tests when the data do not have a normal distribution. In that case the former tests are more sensitive than the latter. They are quick and easy, and are based on ranking of data in their order of magnitude. With heavily skewed data this means that we make the distribution of the ranks look a little bit like a normal distribution. We have paired and unpaired non-parametric tests and with the paired test the same problem of loss of sensitivity with negative correlations is encountered as the one we observed with the paired normality tests as discussed in the preceding paragraph. Non-parametric tests are also used to test normal distributions, and provide hardly different results from their parametric counterparts when distributions are approximately normal. Most frequently used tests:

For paired comparisons:

Mann-Whitney test= **Wilcoxon signed rank** test= **paired Wilcoxon** test

For unpaired comparisons:

Wilcoxon rank sum test

PAIRED TEST: MANN-WHITNEY TEST

Table 10. Paired comparison using Mann-Whitney test: placebo-controlled clinical trial to test efficacy of sleeping drug

	Hours of sleep			rank
Patient	drug	placebo	difference	(ignoring sign)
1	6.1	5.2	0.9	3.5^x
2	7.0	7.9	-0.9	3.5
3.	8.2	3.9	4.3	10
4.	7.6	4.7	2.9	7
5.	6.5	5.3	1.2	5
6.	8.4	5.4	3.0	8
7.	6.9	4.2	2.7	6
8.	6.7	6.1	0.6	2
9.	7.4	3.8	3.6	9
10.	5.8	6.3	-0.5	1

[x]number 3 and 4 in the rank are tight, so we use 3.5 for both of them.

The Mann-Whitney test uses the signs and the relative magnitudes of the data instead of the actual data (table 10). E.g., the above table shows the number of hours sleep in 10 patients tested twice: with sleeping pill and with placebo. We have 3 steps:

1. exclude the differences that are zero, put the remaining differences in ascending order of magnitude and ignore their sign and give them a rank number 1, 2, 3 etc (if differences are equal, average their rank numbers: 3 and 4 become 3.5 and 3.5);

2. add up the positive differences as well as the negative differences;
   + ranknumbers= 3.5+10+7+5+8+6+2+9=50.5
   - ranknumbers= 3.5+1= 4.5

3. The null hypothesis is that there is no difference between += and-ranknumbers. We assess the smaller of the two ranknumbers. The test is significant if the value is smaller than could be expected by chance. We consult the Mann Whitney table showing us the upper values for 5%, and 1% significance, for the number of differences constituting our rank. In this example we have 10 ranks: 5% and 1% points are respectively 8 and 3. The result is significant at $P<0.05$, indicating that the sleeping drug is more effective than the placebo.

UNPAIRED TEST: WILCOXON RANK SUM TEST

Table 11 shows two-samples of patients are treated with 2 different antirheumatic agents. Outcome variable is plasma globulin concentration (g/l). Sample one is printed in standard and sample 2 is printed in fat print.

Table 11.Two-samples of patients are treated with 2 different antirheumatic agents. Outcome variable is plasma globulin concentration (g/l). Sample one is printed in standard and sample 2 is printed in fat print

Globulin concentration(g/l)	ranknumber
26	1
27	**2**
28	3
29	4
30	5
31	6
32	7
33	8
34	**9**
35	10
36	11
38	12.5
38	**12.5**
39	**14.5**
39	**14.5**
40	**16**
41	17
42	**18**
45	**19.5**
45	**19.5**

We have 2 steps:
1. The data from both samples are ranked together in ascending order of magnitude. Equal values are averaged.
2. Add up the rank numbers of each of the two samples. In sample-one we have 81.5, in sample-two we have 128.5. We now can consult the Table for Wilcoxon rank sum test and find with n=10 and n=10 (differences in sample sizes are no problem) that the smaller of the two sums of ranks should be smaller than 71 in order to conclude P<0.05. We can therefore not reject the null hypothesis of no difference, and have to conclude that the two samples are not significantly different from each other.

Note: Kruskall-Wallis test and Friedman test are non parametric tests for analyzing more than two groups and more than two paired observations respectively.

9. REFERENCES

1. Matthews DE, Farewell VT. Using and understanding medical statistics. Karger, Melbourne, Australia, 1996.
2. Cohen A, Posner J. Clinical Drug Research.Kluwer Academic Publishers, Dordrecht, Neth, 1995.
3. Bailar JC, Mosteller F. Medical Uses of Statistics. N Engl J Med Books, Waltham, MA, !986.
4. Swinscow TD. Statistics at square one. BMJ Publishing Group, London, UK, 1996.
5. Glantz SA. Primer of Biostatistics. McGraw-Hill, Singapore, 1992.
6. Motulsky H. Intuitive Statistics. Oxford University Press. New York, 1995.
7. Kuhlmann J, Mrozikiewicz A. What should a clinical pharmacologist know to start a clinical trial? Zuckschwerdt Verlag, Munich, 1998.
8. De Vocht A. SPSS basic guide book. Bijleveld Press, Amsterdam, 1998.
9. Hays WL. Statistics. Holt, Rine and Winston, Toronto, Ontario, 1988.
10. Kirkwood BR. Medical statistics. Blackwell Scientific Publications, Boston, MA, 1990.
11. Petrie A, Sabin C. Medical Statistics at a Glance. Blackwell Science, London, UK, 2000.
12. Riffenburgh RH. Statistics in Medicine. Academic Press. New York, USA, 1999.

CHAPTER 3

THE ANALYSIS OF SAFETY DATA OF DRUG TRIALS

1. INTRODUCTION, SUMMARY DISPLAY

As discussed in chapter 1 the primary object of clinical trials of new drugs is generally to demonstrate efficacy rather than safety. However, a trial in human beings not at the same time adequately addressing safety is unethical, and the assessment of safety variables is an important element of the trial.

An effective approach to the analysis of adverse effects is to present summaries of prevalences. We give an example (table 1). Calculations of the 95% CIs of a proportion is demonstrated in chapter 1. If 0.1<proportion (p) <0.9, the binomial distribution is very close to the normal distribution, but if p < 0.1, the data follow a skewed, otherwise called Poisson distribution. 95 % CIs are, then, more adequately calculated according to $\pm 1.96 \sqrt{p}/n$ rather than $\pm 1.96 \sqrt{p(1-p)}/n$ (confer page 10). Alternatively, tables (e.g., Wissenschaftliche Tabelle, Documenta Geigy, Basel, 1995) and numerous statistical software packages can readily provide you with the CIs.

Table 1. The prevalence of side-effects after 8 week   treatment

side effect	Alpha blocker n=16			alpha plus beta blocker n=15		
	yes	no	95% CIs(%)	yes	no	95% CIs (%)
nasal congestion	10	6	35-85	10	5	38-88
alcohol intolerance	2	12	2-43	2	13	4-71
urine incontinence	5	11	11-59	5	10	12-62
disturbed ejaculation	4	2	22-96	2	2	7-93
disturbed potence	4	2	22-96	2	2	7-93
dry mouth	8	8	25-75	11	4	45-92
tiredness	9	7	30-80	11	4	45-92
palpitations	5	11	11-59	2	13	2-40
dizziness at rest	4	12	7-52	5	10	12-62
dizziness with exercise	8	8	25-75	12	3	52-96
orthostatic dizziness	8	8	25-75	10	5	38-88
sleepiness	5	10	12-62	9	6	32-84

Table 1 gives an example. Numbers relate to the numbers of patients showing a particular side effect. Some questions were not answered by all patients. Particularly, sleepiness occurred differently in the two groups: 33% in the left, 60% in the right group. This difference may be true or due to chance. In order to estimate the size of probability that this difference occurred merely by chance we can perform a statistical test which in case of proportions such is here has to be a chi-square or given the small data a Fisher exact test.

2. FOUR METHODS TO ANALYZE TWO UNPAIRED PROPORTIONS

Using the sleepiness data from above we construct a contingency table

	Sleepiness	no sleepiness
Left treatment (left group)	5 (a)	10 (b)
Right treatment (right group)	9(c)	6 (d)

METHOD-1

Normal test (= z-test for binomial or binary data ≈similar to T-test: T= d/SE , z= d/SE) where d is difference between proportions of sleepers per group.

z = difference between proportions of sleepers per group/
                          standard error of this difference
$z = (5/15 - 9/15) / \sqrt{(SE_1^2 + SE_2^2)}$

SE_1 (or SEM_1) $= p_1 (1-p_1)/ n_1$ where $p_1 = 5/15$ etc.
Reject 0-hypothesis if difference between proportions > 1.96 SEs distant from 0.

METHOD-2

	Sleepiness	no sleepiness
Left treatment (left group)	5 (a)	10 (b)
Right treatment (right group)	9(c)	6 (d)

cell a: $(O-E)^2 / E = (5 - 14/30 \times 15)^2 / 14/30 \times 15 = ..$
"   b: $(O-E)^2 / E$
"   c: $(O-E)^2 / E$
"   d: $(O-E)^2 / E$ _____ +
                                        chi-square = 2.106

(O= observed number; E= expected number=(proportion sleepers /total number) x number$_{group}$).
Reject 0-hypothesis if squared distances from mean > $(1.96)^2$ SEs^2 . We find 2.106 SEs^2 , and, so, the 0-hypothesis can not be rejected.
Note: a chi-square distribution = a squared normal distribution.

METHOD-3

	Sleepiness	no sleepiness	total
Left treatment (left group)	5 (a)	10 (b)	a+b
Right treatment (right group)	9(c)	6 (d)	c+d
	a+c	b+d	

Calculating the chi-square (x^2)- value is calculated according to:

$$\frac{(ad-bc)(a+b+c+d)}{(a+b)(c+d)(b+d)(a+c)}$$

In our case the size of the chi-square is again 2.106 at 1 degree of freedom which means that the 0-hypothesis of no difference not be rejected. The difference is due to chance.

METHOD-4

Fisher-exact test is used for small samples, e.g., samples of n < 100. It, essentially, makes use of faculties expressed as the sign <!>: e.g., 5! indicates 5x4x3x2x1.

	Sleepiness	no sleepiness
Left treatment (left group)	5 (a)	10 (b)
Right treatment (right group)	9(c)	6 (d)

$$P= \frac{(a+b)! ((c+d)! (a+c)! (b+d)!}{(a+b+c+d)! \, a!b!c!d!} = 0.2 \quad \text{(much larger than 0.05)}$$

Again, we can not reject the null-hypothesis of no difference between the two groups. This test is laborious but a computer can calculate the widest faculties for you within 1-2 seconds.

3. CHI-SQUARE TO ANALYZE MORE THAN TWO UNPAIRED PROPORTIONS

Chi-square can be used for multiple tables. The approach is similar to that of above method-2. For example

	Sleepiness	no sleepiness
Group I	5 (a)	10 (b)
Group II	9 (c)	6 (d)
Group III	.. (e)	...(f)
Group IV	..	
Group V		

cell a: $(O-E)^2 / E = (5 - 14/30 \times 15)^2 / 14/30 \times 15 = ..$
    b: $(O-E)^2 / E$
    c: $(O-E)^2 / E$
    d: $(O-E)^2 / E$
    e: ..
    f : ..

$$\overline{\hspace{6cm}} +$$
chi-square = ..

Different is the degrees of freedom: they are 2-1 with 2x2 table, and 5-1 with 5x2 table, etc.

Notes:-Chi-square testing looks weird at first.
      -It is closely related to the normal or T-test.
      -The main difference: it uses squared values.

More details on chi-square statistics and its relationship with other statistical methods are given in chapter 17.

4. MCNEMAR'S TEST FOR PAIRED PROPORTIONS

Paired proportions have to be assessed when e.g. different diagnostic tests are performed in one subject, e.g., 315 subjects are tested for hypertension using an automated device (test-1) and a sphygmomanometer (test-2), (Table 2).

Table 2. Finding discordant pairs

		Test 1		
		+	-	total
Test 2	+	184	54	238
	-	14	63	77
total		198	117	315

$$\text{Chi-square McNemar} = \frac{(54-14)^2}{54+14}$$

184 subjects scored positive with both tests and 63 scored negative with both tests. These 247 subjects therefore give us no information about which of the tests is more likely to score positive. The information we require is entirely contained in the 68 subjects for which tests did not agree (the socalled discordant pairs).

To analyze samples of more than 2 pairs of data, e.g., 3, 4 pairs, etc., McNemar's test can not be applied. For that purpose logistic regression analysis is adequate (chapter 14).

5.SURVIVAL ANALYSIS

SURVIVAL ANALYSIS

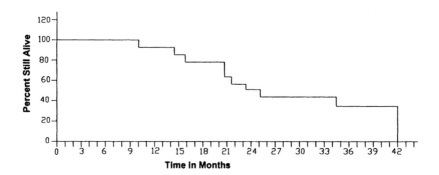

Figure 1. Example of a survival curve plotting survival as a function of time.

A survival curve plots percentage survival as a function of time. Figure 1 is an example. Fifteen patients are followed for 36 months. At time zero everybody is alive. At the end 40% (6/15) patients are still alive. Percentage decreased whenever a patient died. A problem with survival analysis generally is that of lost data: some patients may be still alive at the end of the study but were lost for follow-up for several reasons. We at least know that they lived at the time they were lost, and so they contribute useful information. The data from subjects leaving the study are called **censored** data and should be included.

With the **Kaplan-Meier** method, survival is recalculated every time a patient dies (approaches to survival different from the Kaplan-Meier approach are (1) the actuarial method,where the x-axis is divided into regular intervals and (2) life-table analysis using tables instead of graphs). To calculate the fraction of patients who survive a particular day, simply divide the numbers still alive after the day by the number alive before the day. Also exclude those who are lost=censored on the very day and remove from both the numerator and denominator. To calculate the fraction of patients who survive from day 0 until a particular day, multiply the fraction who survive day-1, times the fraction of those who survive day-2, etc. This product of many survival fractions is called the **product-limit**. In order to calculate the 95% CIs, we can use the formula:

95% CI of the product of survival fractions (p) at time k = p $\pm$ 2. p$\sqrt{(1-p)/k}$

The interpretation: we have measured survival in one sample, and the 95%CI shows we can be 95% sure that the true population survival is within the boundaries (see figure upper and lower boundaries). Instead of days, as time variable, weeks, months etc may be used.

TESTING SIGNIFICANCE OF DIFFERENCE BETWEEN TWO KAPLAN-MEIER CURVES

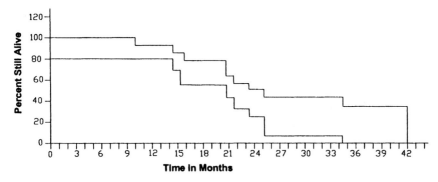

Fig. 2. Kaplan-Meier survival curve with 95% CIs.

Survival is essentially expressed in the form of either proportions or odds, and statistical testing whether one treatment modality scores better than the other in terms of providing better survival can be effectively done by using tests similar to the above **chi-square tests** or chi-square-like tests in order to test whether any proportion of responders is different from another proportion, e.g., the proportion of responders in a control group. RRs or ORs are calculated for that purpose (review chapter 1). For example, in the example in a certain 2-month period we have left the following numbers: a_i and b_i in curve 1, c_i and d_i in curve 2,

Contingency table	Numbers of deaths	numbers alive
Curve 1	a_i	b_i
curve 2	c_i	d_i

$i = 1,2,3,...$

$$\textbf{Odds ratio} = a_i/b_i \ / \ c_i/d_i \ = \ a_id_i/b_ic_i$$

Significance of difference between the curves is calculated according to the added products "ad" divided by "bc". This can be readily carried out by the

Mantel-Haenszl summary chi-square test:

$a_1d_1/n_1 + a_2d_2/n_2 + a_3d_3/n_3 + ... \ / \quad b_1c_1/n_1 + b_2c_2/n_2 + b_3c_3/n_3 ...... = \Sigma(ad/n) \ / \ \Sigma(bc/n)$
where we thus have multiple 2x2 contingency tables e.g. one for every last day of a subsequent month of the study. With 18 months follow-up the procedure would yield 18 2x2-contingency-tables. This Mantel Haenszel summary chi square test is,

when used for comparing survival curves, more routinely called **log rank test** (this name is rather confusing because there is no logarithm involved)

Note: An alternative more sophisticated approach to compare survival curves is the **Cox's proportional hazards model**, a method analogous to **multiple regression analysis** for multiple means of continuous data and to **logistic regression** for proportions in a multivariate model.

6. CONCLUSIONS

In the past two chapters we discussed different statistical methods to test statistically experimental data from clinical trials. We did not emphasize correlation and regression analysis. The point is that correlation and regression analysis test correlations, rather than causal relationships. Two samples may be strongly correlated e.g., two different diagnostic tests for assessment of the same phenomenon. This does ,however, not mean that one diagnostic test causes the other. In testing the data from clinical trials we are mainly interested in causal relationships. When such assessments were statistically analyzed through correlation analyses mainly, we would probably be less convinced of a causal relationship than we are while using prospective hypothesis testing. So, this is the main reason we so far did not address correlation testing extensively. With epidemiological observational research things are essentially different: data are obtained from the observation of populations or the retrospective observation of patients selected because of a particular condition or illness. Conclusions are limited to the establishment of relationships, causal or not. We currently believe that relationships in medical research between a factor and an outcome can only be proven to be causal when between the factor is introduced and subsequently gives rise to the outcome. We are more convinced when such is tested in the form of a controlled clinical trial. A problem with multiple regression and logistic regression analysis as method for analyzing of multiple samples in clinical trials is closely related to this point. There is always an air of uncertainty about such regression data. Many trials use null-hypothesis testing of two variables, and use multiple regression data only to support and enhance the impact of the report, and to make readership more willing to read the report, rather than to prove the endpoints. It is very unsettling to realize that clinicians and clinical investigators often make bold statements about causalities from multivariate analyses. We believe that this point deserves full emphasis, and will therefore address it again in the chapters 8, 9, 14, and 18.

CHAPTER 4

EQUIVALENCE TESTING

1. INTRODUCTION

A study unable to find a difference is not the same as an equivalent study. For example, a study of 3 subjects does not find a significant difference simply because the sample size is too small. Equivalence testing is particularly important for studying the treatment of diseases for which a placebo control would unethical. In the situation a new treatment must be compared with standard treatment. The latter comparison is at risk of finding little differences.

Figure 1 gives an example of a study where the mean result is little different from 0. Is the result equivalent then. H1 represent the distribution of our data and H0 is the null-hypothesis (this approach is more fully explained in chapter 2). What we observe is that the mean of our trial is only 0.9 SEM distant from 0. which is far too little to reject the null-hypothesis. Our result is not significantly different from 0. Whether our result is equivalent to 0, depends on our prior defined criterium of equivalence. In the figure D sets the defined interval of equivalence. If 95% CIs of our trial is completely within this interval, we conclude that equivalence is demonstrated. This mean that with D_1 boundaries we have no equivalence, with D_2 boundaries we do have equivalence. The striped area under curve = the socalled 85 % CIs = the interval approximately between - 2 SEMs and + 2 SEMs (i.e., 1.96 SEMs with normal distributions, a little bit more than 2 SEMs with t-distributions). It is often hard to prior define the D boundaries, but they should be based not on mathematical but rather on clinical arguments, i.e., the boundaries where differences are undisputedly clinically irrelevant.

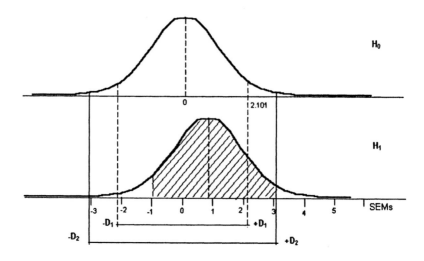

*Figure 1. Null-hypothesis testing and equivalence testing of a
sample of t-distributed data.*

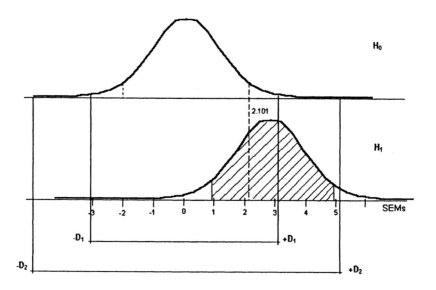

*Figure 2. Null-hypothesis testing and equivalence testing of a
sample of t-distributed data.*

Figure 2 gives another example. The mean result of our trial is larger now: mean
value is 2.9 SEMs distant from 0, and, so, we conclude that the difference from 0

is > approximately 2 SEMs and, that we can reject the null-hypothesis of no difference. Does this mean that our study is not equivalent? This again depends on our prior defined criterium⁻of equivalence. With D_1 the trial is not completely within the boundaries and equivalence is thus not demonstrated. With D_2 the striped area of the trial is completely within the boundaries and we conclude that equivalence has been demonstrated. Note that with D_1 we have both significant difference and equivalence.

2.OVERVIEW OF POSSIBILITIES WITH EQUIVALENCE TESTING

Table 1 shows that any confidence interval (95 % CIs intervals between the brackets in each of the examples) that does not overlap zero is statistically different from zero. Only intervals between the prespecified range of equivalence –D to + D present equivalence. Thus, situations 3, 4 and 5 demonstrate equivalence, while 1 and 2, just like 6 and 7 do not. Situations 3 and 5 present equivalence and at the same time significant difference. Situation 8 presents nor significant difference, nor equivalence.

Table 1. Any confidence interval (95 % CIs intervals between the brackets in each of the examples) that does not overlap zero is statistically different from zero. Only intervals between the prespecified range of equivalence –D to + D present equivalence

Study (1-8)	Statistical significance demonstrated	equivalence demonstrated		
1.	Yes			-------< not equivalent >
2.	Yes			---< uncertain >--------------
3.	Yes		---< equivalent >-------------------------	
4.	No	----< equivalent	>---	
5.	Yes	----< equivalent >-----------------		
6.	Yes	----< uncertain >---		
7.	Yes-< not equivalent >---			
8.	No--------<	uncertain	>--------	

```
                        !                           !
_____
                       -D            O            +D
                               true difference
```

Testing equivalence of two treatments is different from testing their difference. We will in this chapter use the term comparative studies to name the latter kind of studies. In a comparative study we use statistical significance tests to determine whether the null hypothesis of no treatment difference can be rejected, frequently together with 95% CIs to better visualize the size of the difference. In an equivalence study this significance test has little relevance: failure to detect a difference does not imply equivalence; the study may have been too small with corresponding wide standard errors to allow for such a conclusion. Also, not only difference but also equivalence are terms that should be interpreted within the context of clinical relevance. For that purpose we have to predefine a range of equivalence as an interval from –D to +D. We can then simply check whether our 95% CIs as centered on the observed difference lies entirely between –D and +D. If it does equivalence is demonstrated if not, there is room for uncertainty. The above table shows the discrepancies between significance and equivalence testing. The procedure of checking whether the 95% CIs are within a range of equivalence does look somewhat similar to a significance testing procedure, but one in which the role of the usual null and alternative hypothesis are reversed. In equivalence testing the relevant null hypothesis is that a difference of at least D exists, and the analysis is targeted at rejecting this "null hypothesis". The choice of D is difficult, is often chosen on clinical arguments : the new agent should be sufficiently similar to the standard agent to be clinically indistinguishable.

Calculations
95% CIs intervals are calculated according to the standard formulas

Continuous data paired or unpaired and normal distributions (with t-distribution **2**, which is actually 1.96, should be replaced by the appropriate t-value dependent upon sample size).

$$\text{Mean}_1 - \text{mean}_2 \pm \mathbf{2}\ \text{SEMs where}$$
$$\text{SEM}_{\text{unpaired differences}} = \sqrt{(SD_1^2 / n_1 + SD_1^2 / n_2)}$$
$$\text{SEM}_{\text{paired differences}} = \sqrt{(SD_1^2 + SD_2^2 - 2\ r\ SD_1 . SD_2)/n} \quad \text{if } n_1 = n_2 = n$$

Binary data

$$\text{SEM of differences} = \sqrt{p_1/(1-p_1)/ n_1 + p_2/(1-p_2)/ n_2}$$
$$\text{With 95\% CIs :} \quad p_1 - p_2 \pm 2. \text{SEM}$$

More details about the calculation of SEMS of samples are given in chapter 1.
The calculation of required samples size of the trial based on expected treatment effects in order to test our hypothesis reliably, will be explained in the next chapter together with sample size calculations for comparative studies.

It is helpful to present the results of an equivalence study in the form of the a graph (table 1). The result may be:

1. The confidence interval for the difference between the two treatments lies entirely between the equivalence range so that we conclude that equivalence is demonstrated.
2. The confidence interval covers at least several points outside the equivalence range so that we conclude that a clinically important difference remains a possibility, and equivalence cannot be safely concluded.
3. The confidence interval is entirely outside the equivalence range.

3. EQUIVALENCE TESTING, A NEW GOLD STANDARD?

The classic gold standard in drug research is the randomized placebo controlled clinical trial. This design is favored for confirmatory trials as part of the phase III development of new medicines. Because of the large numbers and classes of medicines already available, however, new medicines are increasingly being developed for indications for which a placebo control group would be unethical. In such situations an obvious solution is to use as comparator an existing drug already licensed and regularly used for the indications in question. When an active comparator is used, the expectation may sometimes be that the new treatment will be better than the standard, the objective of the study may be to demonstrate this. This situation would be similar to a placebo control and requires no special methodogy. More probably, however, the new treatment is expected to simply largely match the efficacy of the standard treatment but to have some advantages in terms of safety, adverse effects, costs, pharmacokinetic properties. Under these circumstances the objective of the trial is to show equivalent efficacy.

4.VALIDITY OF EQUIVALENCE TRIALS

A comparative trial is valid when it is blinded, randomized, explicit, accurate statistically and ethically. The same is true for equivalence trial. However, a problem arises with the intention to treat analysis. Intention to treat patients are analyzed according to their randomized treatment irrespective of whether they actually received the treatment. The argument is that it mirrors what will happen when a treatment is used in practice. In a comparative parallel group study the inclusion of protocol violators in the analysis tend to make the results of the two treatments more similar. In an equivalence study this effect may bias the study towards a positive result, being the demonstration of equivalence. A possibility is to carry out both intention-to-treat-analysis and completed-protocol-analysis. If no difference is demonstrated, we conclude that the study's data are robust (otherwise called sensitive, otherwise called precise) , and that the protocol-analysis did not introduce major sloppiness into the data. Sometimes, efficacy and safety endpoints are analyzed differently: the former according to the protocol analysis simply because important endpoint variables are missing in the population that leaves the study early, and intention to treat analysis for the latter, because safety variables frequently include items such as side effects, drop-offs, morbidity and mortality during trial. Either endpoint can of course be assessed in an equivalence assessment trial, but we must consider that an intention to treat analysis may bias the equivalence principle towards overstimation of the chance of equivalence.

Note: statistical power of equivalence testing is explained in the next chapter.

CHAPTER 5

STATISTICAL POWER AND SAMPLE SIZE

1. WHAT IS STATISTICAL POWER

PROBABILITY
DISTRIBUTION

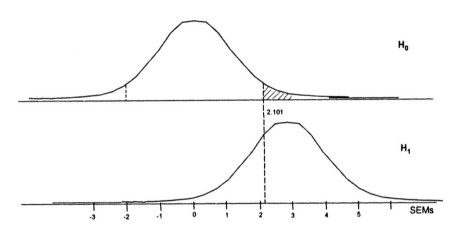

Figure1. H1 is the given distribution with mean value of 2.901 (= t = mean/SEM). β= area under curve (AUC) H1 left from the dotted vertical line= ±0.3 (±30% of the total AUC). 1-β= ±0.7=±70% of total AUC of H1. Statistical power =±0.7=chance of finding a difference when there is one.

Figure 1 shows 2 graphs of t-distributions. The lower graph (H1)could be a probability distribution of a sample of data or of a sample of paired differences between two observations. N=20 and so 95% of the observations is within 2.901 ± 2.101 SEMs on the x-axis (usually called z-axis in statistics). The upper graph is identical, but centers around 0 instead of 2.901. It is called the null hypothesis H0, and represents the data of our sample if the mean results would be not different from zero. However, our mean result is 2.901 SEMs distant from zero. If we had many samples obtained by similar trials under the same null hypothesis, the chance of finding a mean value of more than 2.101 is < 5%, because the area under the curve (AUC) of H0 right from 2.101 <5% of total AUC. We, therefore, reject the assumption that our results indicate a difference just by chance and decide that we have demonstrated a true difference. What is the power of this test. The power has as prior assumption that there is a difference from zero in our data. What is the chance of demonstrating a difference if there is one. If our experiment would be performed many times, the distribution of obtained mean values of those many experiments would center around 2.901, and about 70% of the AUC of H1 would be larger than 2.101. When smaller than 2.101, our statistical analysis would not be able to reject the null hypothesis of no difference, when larger, it would rightly be able to reject the null hypothesis of no difference. So, in fact 100-70=30% of the many trials would erroneously be unable to reject the null hypothesis of no difference, even when a true difference is in the data. We say the power of this experiment= 1-0.3=0.7 (70%), otherwise called the chance of finding a difference when there is one (area under curve $(1-\beta)$x 100%). β is also called the chance of making a type 2 error= chance of finding no difference when there is one. Another chance is the chance of finding a difference when there is none, otherwise called the type I error (area under the curve $(2x\ \alpha/2)$x 100%). This type of error is usually set to be 0.05 (5%).

2. EMPHASIS ON STATISTICAL POWER RATHER THAN NULL-HYPOTHESIS TESTING

Generally, statistical tests reach their conclusions by seeing how compatible the observations were with the null hypothesis of no treatment effect or treatment difference between test-treatment and reference-treatment. In any test we reject the null hypothesis of no treatment effect if the value of the test statistic (F, t, q, or chi-square) was bigger than 95% of the values that would occur if the treatment had no effect. When this is so, it is common for medical investigators to report a statistically significant effect at P (probability) <0.05 which means that the chance of finding no difference if there is one, is less than 5%. On the other hand, when the test statistic is not big enough to reject this null hypothesis of no treatment effect, the investigators often report no statistically significant difference and discuss their results in terms of documented proof that the treatment had no effect. All they really did, was fail to demonstrate that it did have an effect. The distinction between positively demonstrating that a treatment had no effect and failing to demonstrate that it does have an effect, is subtle but very important, especially with respect to the small numbers of subjects usually enrolled in a trial. A study of treatments that involves only a few subjects and then fails to reject the null hypothesis of no treatment effect, may arrive at this result because the statistical procedure lacked power to detect the effect because of a too small sample size, even though the treatment did have an effect.

PROBABILITY
DISTRIBUTION

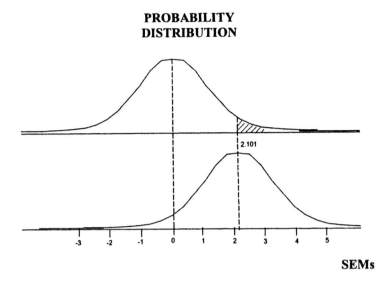

SEMs

Figure 2.   Example of t-distribution with n=20 and its null hypothesis of no effect. Lower curve H1 or actual SEM distribution of the data, upper curve H0 or null hypothesis of the study.

Figure 2 gives an example of a t-distribution with n=20 (H1) and its null hypothesis of no effect (H0). 95% of all similar trials with no significant treatment difference from zero must have their means between –2.101 and +2.101 SEMs from zero. The chance of finding a mean value of 2.101 SEMs or more is 5% or less (α= 0.05 or α. 100%= 5%, where α is the chance of finding a difference when there is none= erroneously rejecting the null hypothesis of no effect, also called type I error). The figure shows that in this particular situation the chance of β is 0.5 or β times 100% = 50% (β is the chance of finding no difference where there is one= the chance of erroneously accepting the null hypothesis of no treatment difference, also called type II error).

Statistical power, defined as 1-β, can be best described as the chance of finding a difference where there is one= the chance of rightly rejecting the null hypothesis of no effect. The figure shows that this chance of detecting a true-positive effect, i.e., reporting a statistically significant difference when the treatment really produces an effect is only 50%, and likewise that the chance of no statistically significant difference is no less than 50% either (β=0.5). It means that if we reject the null hypothesis of no effect at P=0.05, we still have a chance of 50% that a real effect in our data is not detected. As a real effect in the data rather than no effect is the main underlying hypothesis of comparative drug trials, a 50% chance to detect it, is hardly acceptable for reliable testing. A more adequate cut-off level of rejecting would be, e.g., a 90-95% power level, with corresponding α level of 0.005 to

0.001. Many physicians and even some investigators never confront these problems because they never heard of power. An additional advantage of power analysis is the possibility to use power computations on hypothesized results a priori in order to decide on sample size for a study in advance.

3. POWER COMPUTATIONS

Calculating power can be best left over to a computer, because other approaches are rather unprecise. E.g., with normal or t-distributions power $=1-\beta$ can be readily visualized from a graph as estimated percentage of the $(1-\beta)$ x 100% area under the curve. However, errors as large as 10-20 % are unavoidable with this approach. We may alternatively use tables for t- and z-distributions, but as tables give discrete values this procedure is rather inaccurate either.
A computer will make use of the following equations.

For t-distributions of continuous data
Power = $1-\beta$= 1- probability $[z_{power} \leq (t^{1}-t)]$ = probability $[z_{power} >(t^{1}-t)]$

where z_{power} represents a fragment on the x-axis of the z-distribution(or in this particular situation more correctly t-distribution), and t^{1} represents the level of t that for the given degrees of freedom ($\approx$ sample size) yields an α of 0.05. Finally, t in the equation is the actual t as calculated from the data.
Let's assume we have a parallel-group data comparison with test statistic of t=3.99 and n=20 (P<0.001). What is the power of this test? Z_{power} = $(t^{1}-t)$= 3.99-2.101=1.89. This is so, because t^{1}= the t that with dfs 18 (n= 20, 20-2) yields an α of 0.05. To convert z_{power} into power we look up in the t-table with dfs=18 the closest level of probability and find approximately 0.9 for 1.729. The power of this test thus is approximately 90%.

For proportions
z_{power}= 2. (arcsine $\sqrt{p_1}$- arcsine $\sqrt{p_2}$)$\sqrt{n/2}$ - z^{1}

where z_{power} is a fragment of the x-axis of the z-distribution and z^{1} is 2 if α=0.05 (actually 1.96). It is surprising that arcsine (= 1/sine) expressed in rads shows up but it turns out that power is a function of the square roots of the proportions.
A computer turns z_{power} into power. Actually, power graphs as presented in many current texts on statistics can give acceptable estimates for proportions as well.

For equivalence testing of samples with t-distributions and continuous data
Power= $1-\beta$= 1- probability $[z< (D/SEM - z_{1-\alpha})]$
where z is again a fragment on x-axis of the z- or t-distribution and SEM is the square root of the variance of the treatment comparison and $z_{1-\alpha}$ is 2 , actually 1.96.

4. EXAMPLE OF POWER COMPUTATION USING THE T-TABLE

Although a table gives discrete values, and is somewhat inaccurate to precisely calculate the power size, it is useful to master the method, because it is helpful to understand what statistical power really is. The example of Figure 3 is given. Our trial mean is 2.878 SEMs distant from 0 (=the t-value of our trial). We will try to find beta by subtracting T-T^1 where T^1 is the T that yields an area under the curve (AUC) of 5%= 2.101. T-T^1= 2.878-2.101=0.668. Now we can use the t-table to find 1-beta= power.

PROBABILITY
DISTRIBUTION

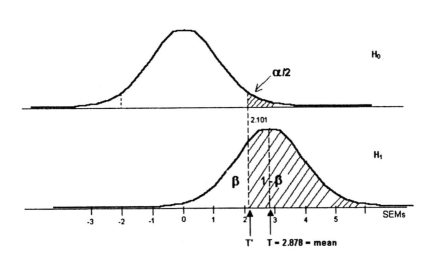

Figure 3. Example of power computation using the t-table.

The t-table gives 8 columns of t-values and one column (left one) of degrees of freedom. The upper rows give an overview of AUCs corresponding to various t-values and degrees of freedom. In our case we have two groups of 10 subjects and thus 20-2=18 degrees of freedom. The AUC right from 2.101 = 0.05 (tested 2-sided= tested for both >+2.101 and <-2.101 distant from 0). Now for the power analysis. The t-value of our trial = approximately 2.9. T^1 = approximately 2.1. T-T^1 = approximately 0.68. The AUC right from 0.688= 0.25= 25%, which is beta (always tested one-sided), and, so, 1-beta = 1-0.25 = 0.75 = 75%.

T-Table: v= degrees of freedom for t-variable, Q=proportion of cases cut off on the upper tail of the t- distribution

v	Q = 0.4	0.25	0.1	0.05	0.025	0.01	0.005	0.001
	2Q = 0.8	0.5	0.2	0.1	0.05	0.02	0.01	0.002
1	0.325	1. 000	3.078	6.314	12.706	31.821	63.657	318.31
2	.289	0.816	1.886	2.920	4.303	6.965	9.925	22.326
3	.277	.765	1.638	2.353	3.182	4.547	5.841	10.213
4	.171	.741	1.533	2.132	2.776	3.747	4.604	7.173
5	0.267	0.727	1.476	2.015	2.571	3.365	4.032	5.893
6	.265	.718	1.440	1.943	2.447	3.143	3.707	5.208
7	.263	.711	1.415	1.895	2.365	2.998	3.499	4.785
8	.262	.706	1.397	1.860	2.306	2.896	3.355	4.501
9	.261	.703	1.383	1.833	2.262	2.821	3.250	4.297
10	0.261	0. 700	1.372	1.812	2.228	2.764	3.169	4.144
11	.269	.697	1.363	1.796	2.201	2.718	3.106	4.025
12	.269	.695	1.356	1.782	2.179	2.681	3.055	3.930
13	.259	.694	1.350	1.771	2.160	2.650	3.012	3.852
14	.258	.692	1.345	1.761	2.145	2.624	2.977	3.787
15	0.258	0.691	1.341	1.753	2.131	2.602	2.947	3.733
16	.258	.690	1.337	1.746	2.120	2.583	2.921	3.686
17	.257	.689	1.333	1.740	2.110	2.567	2.898	3.646
18	.257	688	1.330	1.734	2.101	2.552	2.878	3.610
19	.257	.688	1.328	1.729	2.093	2.539	2.861	3.579
20	0.257	0.687	1.325	1.725	2.086	2.528	2.845	3.552
21	.257	.686	1.323	1.721	2.080	2.518	2.831	3.527
22	.256	.686	1.321	1.717	2.074	2.508	2.819	3.505
23	.256	.685	1.319	1.714	2.069	2.600	2.807	3.485
24	.256	.685	1.318	1.711	2.064	2.492	2.797	3.467
25	0.256	0.684	1,316	1.708	2.060	2.485	2.787	3.450
26	.256	.654	1,315	1.706	2.056	2.479	2.779	3.435
27	.256	.684	1,314	1.701	2.052	2.473	2.771	3.421
28	.256	.683	1,313	1.701	2.048	2.467	2.763	3.408
29	.256	.683	1.311	1.699	2.045	2.462	2.756	3.396
30	0.256	0.683	1.310	1.697	2.042	2.457	2.750	3.385
40	.255	.681	1.303	1.684	2.021	2.423	2.704	3.307
60	.254	.679	1.296	1.671	2.000	2.390	2.660	3.232
120	.254	.677	1.289	1.658	1.950	2.358	2.617	3.160
∞	.253	.674	1.282	1.645	1.960	2.326	2.576	3.090

5. CALCULATION OF REQUIRED SAMPLE SIZE, RATIONALE

An essential part of planning a clinical trial is to decide how many people need to be studied in order to answer the study objectives. Just pulling the sample sizes out of a hat gives rise to:

1. Ethical problems, because if too many patients are given a potentially inferior treatment, this is not ethical to do.
2. Scientific problems, because negative studies require the repetition of the research.
3. Financial problems, because extra costs are involved too small and too large studies.

If we have no prior arguments to predict the outcome of a trial, we at least will have an idea of the kind of result that would be clinically relevant. This is also a very good basis to place prior sample size requirement on. A smaller study, for example, will be needed to detect a fourfold increase than a twofold one. So the sample size also depends on the size of result we want to demonstrate reliably.

6. CALCULATIONS OF REQUIRED SAMPLE SIZE, METHODS

Essential part of planning a clinical trial is to decide: how many people need to be studied in order to answer the study objectives.

A simple method :
Mean should be at least 1.96 or approximately 2 SEMs distant from 0 to obtain statistical significance.
Assume: mean = 2 SEM
Then   mean/ SEM=2
Then   mean/ SD/ $\sqrt{n}$ = 2
Then $\sqrt{n}$= 2.SD/mean
Then   **n= 4. (SD/mean)^2**
For example, with mean=10 and SD=20 we will need a sample size of at least n= 4 $(20/10)^2$ = 4 x 4 = **16**. P-value is then 0.05 but power is only 50%.

A more accurate method is the power index method:
The statistical power (1) of a trial assessing a new treatment vs control is determined by 3 major variables:
(2)   D (mean difference or mean result),
(3)   Variance in the data estimated as SD or SEM,
(4)   Sample size.
It follows that we can calculate (4) if we know the other 3 variables.
The relationship between (4) and the 3 other variables can be expressed in fancy formulas with $(z_\alpha + z_\beta)^2$ = **power index** as an important element in all of them. Here is the formula for continuous variables

$$n = 2. (SD/mean)^2 (z_\alpha + z_\beta)^2$$

If power index for null hypothesis is $(z_\alpha + z_\beta)^2$, what is the size of this $(z_\alpha + z_\beta)^2$?

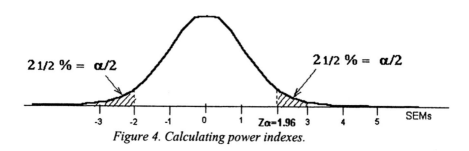

Figure 4. Calculating power indexes.

What does for example $Z_{(alpha)}$ exactly mean? $Z_{(alpha)}$ **means " a place" on the Z-line. What place?** If alpha is defined 5%, or rather 2x2 1/2 % , then right from this place on the Z-line AUC = 5%, or rather 2x2 1/2 %. So this place must be 1.96 SEMs distant from 0, or a bit more with t-distribution. **So Z_{alpha} = 1.96= approximately 2.0** (Figure 4).

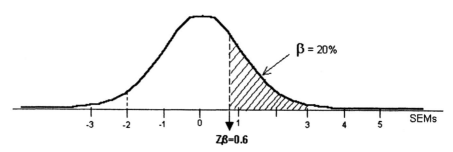

Figure 5. Calculating power indexes.

What does $Z_{(beta)}$ exactly mean? If **beta** is defined 20%, what is the place on Z-line of $Z_{(beta)}$? Right from this place the AUC= 20% of the total AUC. This means that this place must be approximately 0.6 SEMs distant from 0. **So Z $_{beta}$ = approximately 0.6** (Figure 5).

Now we can calculate the power index $(z_\alpha + z_\beta)^2$.

$Z_{(alpha)}$ = approximately 2.0
$Z_{(beta)}$ = approximately 0.6
power index = $(z_\alpha + z_\beta)^2 = 2.6^2 = 6.4$
As the formula for continuous variables n= 2. $(SD/mean)^2 (z_\alpha + z_\beta)^2$
, we can now conclude that with α = 5% and power = 1- β = 80% the required
sample size is n= 12.8 $(SD/mean)^2$. E.g., with SD=20 and mean=10 we will need a
sample size of n= 12.8 (20/ 10)^2 = **51.**
**So accounting a power of 80% requires 51 rather than the 16 patients
required according to the simple method.**

Other formulas for sample size computations include:

Required sample size formula for proportions
$N= 2\ p_{average} (1- p_{average}) (z_\alpha + z_\beta)^2\ / D^2$

Required sample size formula for equivalence testing
$N = 2$ **(between subject variance)** $(z_{1-1/2\alpha} + z_{1-1/2\beta})^2 / D^2$
(where D is minimal difference we wish to detect).

What size is **power index of equivalence test** $(z_{1-1/2\alpha} + z_{1-1/2\beta})^2$?
If power index of equivalence testing $= (z_{1-1/2\alpha} + z_{1-1/2\beta})^2$
What is the size of this power index?

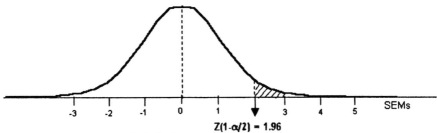

Z(1-α/2) = 1.96
Figure 6. Calculating power indexes.

If alpha is defined 5%, then ½ alpha = 2 ½ %. What is the place on the Z-line of Z
$_{(1-1/2\alpha)}$? **Left from this place is the AUC = 1- ½ alpha = 100- 2 ½ %= 97 ½ %
of total AUC.** So this place is, just like Z_{alpha} , 1.96 SEMs distant from 0, or bit
more with t-distribution. So, $Z_{(1- ½\ alpha)}$ = **1.96 or approximately 2.0** (Figure 6).

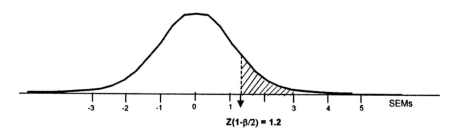

$$Z(1-\beta/2) = 1.2$$

Figure 7. Calculating power indexes.

Now, if beta is defined 20%, then ½ beta = 10% What is the place on the Z-line of $Z_{(1-1/2\ beta)}$? **Left from the place the AUC = 100% -10% = 90% of total AUC.** This means that this place must be app 1.2 SEMs distant from 0, or bit more. So $Z_{(1-\frac{1}{2}\ beta)}$ = **approximately 1.2** (Figure 7).

Now we can calculate this power index. So $Z_{(1-\frac{1}{2}\alpha)}$ = app 2.0. $Z_{(1-\frac{1}{2}\beta)}$ = app 1.2. The power index for equivalence testing = $(2.0 + 1.2)^2$ = approximately 10.9.

NOTE: power index null hypothesis testing =   6.4
          "   "   equivalence testing = 10.9

Obviously, for equivalence testing larger sample sizes are required !

Equivalence trials often include too few patients. The conclusion of equivalence becomes meaningless if, due to this, the design lacks power. Testing equivalence usually requires a sample at least twice that of comparative null hypothesis testing studies. Required numbers of patients to be included should be estimated at the design stage of such studies.

7. TESTING NOT ONLY SUPERIORITY BUT ALSO INFERIORITY OF A NEW TREATMENT (THE TYPE III ERROR)

An inferior treatment may sometimes mistakingly be believed to be superior. "Negative"studies, defined as studies that do not confirm their prior hypotheses, may be "negative"because an inferior treatment is mistakingly believed to be superior. However, from a statistical point of view this possibility is unlikely. Suppose in a study the mean results is + 1 SEM distant from the mean of the null hypothesis of no treatment effect (Figure 8).

PROBABILITY
DISTRIBUTION

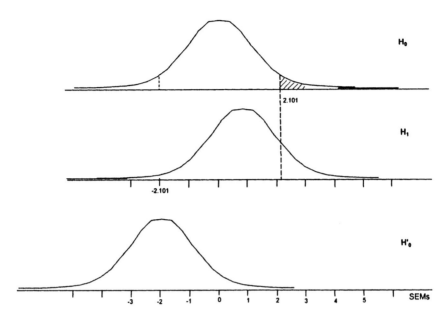

Figure 8. Study with n=20 and mean results + 1 SEM distant from the mean of the null hypothesis of no treatment effect. For testing the chance that our treatment is significantly inferior, a new null hypothesis at approximately – 2SEMs distant from zero is required.

This means that we are unable to reject this null hypothesis, because a null hypothesis is rejected when the mean result of a study is more than about 2 SEMs distant from zero (P<0.05), and the study is thus "negative". For testing the chance that our treatment is significantly inferior, a new null hypothesis at approximately – 2SEMs distant from zero is required. This null hypothesis is about 3 SEMs distant from our mean result, which means that this chance is <0.001. So, it seems that even statistically "negative"trials give strong evidence that the favored treatment is, indeed, not inferior. This issue can be illustrated by an example. The treatment of hypertension is believed to follow a J-shape curve, where overtreatment produces increased rather than reduced mortality/morbidity. A different theory would tell you that the more intensive the therapy the better the result. This latter theory was recently tested in the HOT trial[1] (HOT investigators, Lancet 1998; 87: 133), but could not be confirmed: high dosage antihypertensive therapy was not significantly better than medium-dosage therapy. Probably it was not worse either, however, unfortunately, this was not tested in the report. The study would definitely have been powerful to test this question, and, moreover, it would have solved a major so far unsolved discussion.

An additional advantage of testing type III errors is that it helps preventing well-designed studies from going down in history as just "negative"studies that did not prove anything and are more likely not to be published, leading to unnecessary and costly repetition of research. If such socalled "negative"studies are capable of rejecting the chance of a type III error, they may be reconsidered as a study that is not completely negative and may be rightly given better priority for being published.

8. REFERENCES

1.   HOT investigators. The HOT trial. Lancet 1998; 87: 133.

CHAPTER 6

INTERIM ANALYSES

1. INTRODUCTION

Clinical trials tend to have a long duration, because mostly patients are enrolled one by one, and their responses to treatment are observed sequentially. For the organizers this part of the trial is an exciting phase because after all the hard work involved in planning and getting the trial started, finally concrete data will become available. Immediately, there is the possibility to look at the data in order to check that the trial protocol is pursued appropriately by the investigators and to look at any difficulties, e.g., those with patient and/or doctor compliance, and to see whether there is any need for protocol alterations[1]. "Looking at the data" for such purposes should, however, be done carefully. In this chapter we will discuss questions such as:
1.   why should we monitor a trial;
2.   who should monitor a trial;
3.   what should be monitored;
4.   why should we be careful.

2. MONITORING

Careful conduct of a clinical trial according to the protocol has a major impact on the credibility of the results[2]; to ensure patient/doctor compliance with the protocol, careful monitoring of the trial is a prerequisite. In large-scale pharmaceutical phase III trials, mainly two types of monitoring are being used: one is concerned with quality assessment of trial, and the other with the assumptions that were made in the protocol concerning treatment differences, power, and adverse effects. The quality of the trial is greatly enhanced when checks are performed to ensure that

1.   the protocol requirements are appropriately met by investigators and patients;
2.   inclusion and exclusion criteria are appropriately met;
3.   the rate of inclusion of patients in the trial is in accordance with the trial plan;
4.   the data are being accrued properly, and;
5.   design assumptions are met.

This type of monitoring does not require access to the data in the trial, nor is unblinding necessary, and therefore has no impact on the Type I error of finding a difference where there is none[2] (see also chapter 5.1, and 5.2 of the current book).

Usually, this type of monitoring is carried out by a specialized monitoring team under the responsibility of the steering committee of the trial. The period for this type of monitoring starts with the selection of the trial centers and ends with the collection and cleaning of the last patient's data.

Inclusion and exclusion criteria should be kept constant, as specified in the protocol, throughout the period of patient recruitment. In very long-term trials accumulating medical knowledge either from outside the trial, or from interim analyses, may warrant a change in inclusion or exclusion criteria. Also, very low recruitment rates due to over-restrictive criteria, may sometimes favor some change in the criteria. These should be made without breaking the blinding of the trial and should always be described in a protocol amendment to be submitted to the ethic committee for their approval. This amendment should also cover any statistical consequences such as sample size, and alterations to the planned statistical analysis.

The rate of subject accrual should be monitored carefully, especially with long-term trials. If it falls below the expected level, the reasons why so should be identified, and action taken not to jeopardize the power of the trial. Naturally, the quality of the data should be assessed carefully. Attempts should be made to recover missing data and to check the consistency of the data.

3. INTERIM ANALYSIS

The other type of monitoring requires the comparison of treatment results, and it, therefore, generally requires at least partly unblinded access to treatment group assignment. This type of monitoring is actually called interim analysis. It refers to any analysis intended to compare treatment arms with respect to efficacy or safety at any time prior to formal completion of the trial.

The primary goals for monitoring trial data through interim analysis include

1.   ethical concerns to avoid any patient receiving a treatment the very moment it is recognized to be inferior;
2.   (cost-)efficiency concerns of avoiding undue prolongation of a trial once the treatment differences are reasonably clear-cut, and;
3.   checking whether prior assumptions concerning sample size, treatment efficacy and adverse effects are still valid.

As the sample-size of the trial is generally based on preliminary and/or uncertain information, an interim check on the unblinded data may also be useful to reveal whether or not overall response variances, event rates or survival experience are as anticipated. A revised sample size may then be required using suitable modified assumptions. As a matter of course, such modification should be documented in a protocol amendment and in the clinical study report. Steps taken to preserve blindness during the rest of the trial and consequences for the risk of type I errors and the width of the confidence intervals should be accounted for.

Particularly, severe toxic reactions, as well as other adverse effects, are important and need careful observation and reporting to the steering committee, so that prompt action can be taken. Investigators need to be warned to look out for such events and dose modifications may be necessary.

Every process of examining and analyzing data as accumulated in a clinical trial, either formally or informally, can introduce bias and/or increase of type I errors. Therefore, all interim analyses, formal or informal, preplanned or ad hoc, by any study participant, steering committee member, or data monitoring group should be described in full in the clinical study report, even if their results were disclosed to the investigators while on trial[3].

For the purpose of reducing the risk of biases there are a number of important points in the organisation of the analysis and the interpretation of its results to keep in mind.

I - In most trials there are many outcome variables, but in interim analyses it is best to limit the number to only the major variables in order to avoid the multiple comparison problem
(referred to in chapter 1.1). Pocock[1] recommends to use only one main treatment comparison for which a formal 'stopping rule' may be defined, and to use the other treatment comparisons only as an informal check on the consistency of any apparent difference in the main comparison.

II - It is important to perform the interim analysis on correct and up-to-date data. The data monitoring and data checks should be performed on all of the data generated at the time of the interim analysis in order to avoid any selection bias in the patients.

III - The interim analysis should be performed only when there is a sufficient number of patients. Any comparison is academic when the sample size is so small that even huge treatment differences will not be significant.

IV - The interim analysis should not be too elaborate, because there is a limited goal, namely to check whether differences in the main treatment comparison are not huge to the extent that further continuation of the trial would seem unethical.

V - The interim analysis should be planned only when a decision to stop the trial is a serious possibility. With very long-term treatment periods in a trial when the period between patient entry and observance of patient outcome is very long, the patient accrual may be completed before any interim analysis can be performed and the interim analysis results will have no impact on the trial anymore.

VI - The decision to stop the trial must be made according to a predefined stopping rule. The rule should be formulated in terms of magnitude and statistical significance of treatment differences and must be considered in the light of adverse effects, current knowledge, and practical aspects such as ease of administration, acceptability and cost. We must decide in advance what evidence of a treatment difference is sufficiently strong to merit stopping the trial. Statistical significance is a commonly used criterium, but the usual P-level is not appropriate. The problem with statistical significance testing of interim data is that the risk of a type I error may be considerably increased because we perform more than one analysis. Hence, for a sequence of interim analyses we must set a more stringent significance level than the usual P<0.05. We may use a bonferroni adjustment (see also chapter 1 introduction), i.e., use as significance level the value 0.05 divided by the number of planned interim analyses, but this leads in most cases to a somewhat overconservative significance level. Therefore, in most trials a so-called group-sequential design is employed. This subject will be discussed in the next section. A practical guideline is to use Pocock's criteria [4]: **if one anticipates no more than 10 interim analyses and there is one main response variable, one can adopt P<0.01 as the criterion for stopping the trial.** An example of this approach is the following: "stop the trial if the treatment difference is 20% or larger and this difference is statistically significant with a P-value less than 0.01, and the proportion patients with adverse effects is less than 10%." The outcome of the interim analysis may also be such that the treatments differ far less than expected. In such case the trial might be stopped for lack of efficacy. Again, it is essential that a formal stopping rule is formulated in advance specifying the boundary for the treatment difference for the given CIs. In this case statistical significance is not helpful as an additional criterion, but it is helpful to calculate the confidence interval of the observed treatment difference and to see whether the expected treatment difference, specified in the protocol, is far outside that interval.

VII - It is necessary to keep the results of the interim analysis as confidential as possible. Investigators may change their outlook and future participation to the trial, and might even change their attitudes towards treatment of patients in the trial if he/she is aware of any interim results. This may cause a serious bias to the overall trial results. The U.S. Food and Drug Administration (FDA) therefore recommends not only that the execution of the interim analysis be highly confidential[2], but also that the investigators not be informed about its results unless a decision to stop the trial has been made. An external independent group of investigators should ideally perform the interim analysis, for the benefit of the objectivity of the research (although complete independence may be an illusion, it is still better to have some other persons with their own ethical and scientific principles look at your data than do it yourself). The steering committee should be informed about the decisions to continue or discontinue or the implementation of protocol amendments only.

VIII - There is little advantage to be gained from carrying out a large number of interim analyses: the consequences of executing many interim analyses are that the sample sizes are small (at least in the first analyses), and that a smaller significance level must be used. Pocock[5] recommends never to plan more than 5 interim analyses, but at the same time to plan at least one interim analysis, in order to warrant scientific and ethical validity of the trial.

4. GROUP-SEQUENTIAL DESIGN OF INTERIM ANALYSIS

Group sequential design is the most widely used method to define the stopping rule precisely and it was introduced by Pocock.[7] The FDA[2] advocates the use of this design, though it is not the only acceptable type of design, and the FDA does so particularly for the purpose of safety assessment, one of its major concerns.

In a group-sequential trial we need to decide about the number (N) of interim analyses and the number (n) of patients per treatment that should be evaluated in between successive analyses: i.e. if the trial consists of two treatment arms 2n patients must be evaluated in each interim analysis. Pocock[7] (and extensively explained in Pocock[3] provides tables for the exact nominal significance levels depending on the number of interim analyses N and the overall significance level ,. For instance if a trial is evaluated using a normal distributed response variable with known variance and one wishes the overall significance level to be ,=0.05 and one plans N=2 analyses, then the nominal significance level must be set at 0.0294. If N=3 or 4 or 5, the nominal significance levels must be set at 0.0221, 0.0182, and 0.0158, respectively. For other types of response variables, Pocock[7] provides similar tables. Pocock[7] also provides tables of the optimal sample size numbers of patients to be included in successive interim analyses.

Several extensions of the practical rules of Pocock were developed, for instance rules for letting the nominal significance level vary between interim analyses. In practice a far more stringent p-value is suggested for earlier interim analyses and a less stringent one for later analyses. Pocock[1] claimed that such a variation might be sensible for studies with a low power, but that almost no efficiency is gained in studies with powers of 90% or higher. Other extensions concern one-sided testing[8] and skewed designs where a less stringent rule might be adopted for stopping if the new treatment is worse than the standard and a more stringent rule if the new treatment appears to be better than the standard.

5. CONTINUOUS SEQUENTIAL STATISTICAL TECHNIQUES

Historically, the statistical theory for stopping rules in clinical trials has been largely concerned with sequential designs for continuous monitoring of treatment differences. The basic principle is that after every additional patient on each treatment has been evaluated, some formal statistical rule is applied to the whole data so far to determine whether the trial should stop. The theory of sequential techniques is already quite old (developed in the early fourties and even earlier than that[9]), and many excellent textbooks have been published[10]; here we adopt the arguments of Whitehead.[11]

The central idea is to calculate after each additional patient (or after I additional patients) (a function of) the treatment difference, called Z, and the total amount of information, called V, sampled thus far. These two statistics are plotted graphically against each other each time a new patient is evaluated. The stopping rule of the trial entails evaluating whether a boundary is crossed. In Figure 1 a typical example of a sequential trial with a so-called triangular test is illustrated.

Treatment difference (z)

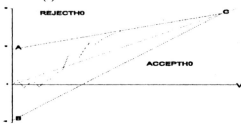

Total amount of information(v)

Figure 1. Typical example of a sequential trial with a so-called triangular test.
The undulating line illustrates a possible realisation of a clinical trial: after each
time a new patient could be evaluated, Z and V are calculated and the line is
extended a little further. The line-sections AC and BC are the stopping boundaries,
and the triangular region ABC is the continuation region. If the sample path crosses
AC, the null hypothesis is rejected at the 5% significance level, and if BC is crossed
then H₀ is accepted. When Z is replaced by t or chi-square statistic, and V by degrees
of freedom, the graph represents very much the same as the t- or chi-square tables
(appendix) respectively do.

The undulating line illustrates a possible realisation of a clinical trial: after each time a
new patient could be evaluated, Z and V are calculated and the line is extended a little
further. The line-sections AC and BC are the stopping boundaries, and the triangular
region ABC is the continuation region. If the sample path crosses AC, the null
hypothesis is rejected at the 5% significance level, and if BC is crossed then H_0 is
accepted. The triangular test is one of many possible sequential trial designs; but the
triangular test has some very attractive characteristics. If the treatment difference is
large, it will lead to a steeply increasing sample path, and consequently to a small trial
because the AC boundary is reached quickly. If there is no difference between
treatment, the sample path will move horizontally and will cross the BC boundary
quickly which also leads to a small trial. If the treatment difference is negative, the BC
boundary will be crossed even quicker.
The trick is to devise sensible boundaries. Whitehead [11] gives an elaborate discussion
on how to do this (as well as how to calculate Z and V). Whitehead [11] also discussed
many different sequential plans for many different types of clinical trials and data-
types. Whitehead and his associates have also developed a user-friendly computer
program to design and analyze sequential clinical trials. [12]

6. CONCLUSIONS

Interim analyses in clinical trials can be of great importance in maintaining quality standards of the entire investigation and such analyses may be of crucial importance if clinical trials are to be ethically acceptable. Drawbacks of interim analyses are the increased risk of the type I error and the potential introduction of several kinds of biases, such as loss of validity factors, including blinding and randomization . It is rarely sensible to perform more than 5 interim analyses and usual 1 interim analysis before the final assessment suffices. It is crucial to specify in advance in the study protocol, how many analyses are to be performed and on how many patients, and which decisions are to be made on the basis of the interim results. It is best to let an external independent group, often called Independent Data Monitoring Committee (IDMC), execute the job and to keep its results as confident as is ethically possible. To do so, will be difficult but rewarding, and contribute to the credibility and scientific value of the trial results.

7. REFERENCES

1. Pocock SJ. Clinical trials. A practical approach. New York: Wiley, 1988.
2. Department of Health and Human Services, Food and Drug Administration. International Conference on Harmonisation; Guidance on Statistical Principles for Clinical Trials Availability. Federal Register, 63 (179), 1998: 49583-49598.
3. Food and Drug Administration. Guideline for Industry. Structure and Content of Clinical Study reports. FDA, 1996: at internet webside WWW.DFA.GOV /CDER/REGGUIDE.HTM/GUIDANCE DOCUMENTS.
4. Pocock SJ. Clinical trials. A practical approach. New York: Wiley, 1988, page 147.
5. Pocock SJ. Clinical trials. A practical approach. New York: Wiley, 1988, page 153.
6. Pocock SJ. Clinical trials. A practical approach. New York: Wiley, 1988, page 149.
7. Pocock SJ. Group sequential methods in the design and analysis of clinical trials. Biometrika 1977; 64: 191-199.
8. Demets DL, Ware JH. Group sequential methods in clinical trials with a one-sided hypothesis. Biometrika, 1980, 67: 651-660.
9. Wald A. Sequential Analysis. New York: Wiley, 1947.
10. Armitage P. Sequential Medical Trials. Oxford: Blackwell, 1975.
11. Whitehead J. The design and analysis of sequential clinical trials. Chichester: Ellis Horwood publishers, 1983.
12. Whitehead J. Planning and Evaluating Sequential Trials (PEST, version 3). Reading: University of Reading, 1998 (www.reading.ac.uk/mps/pest/pest.html)

CHAPTER 7

MULTIPLE STATISTICAL INFERENCES

1. INTRODUCTION

Clinical trials often compare the efficacy of several new treatments and often use many efficacy variables. Also, after overall testing for significant differences, additional questions about subgroups differences or about what variables do or do not contribute to the efficacy results. Assessment of such questions introduces the statistical problem of multiple comparison and multiple testing, which increases the risk of false positive statistical results, and thus increases the type-I error risk. In this chapter simple methods are discussed which can help to control this risk.

2. MULTIPLE COMPARISONS

When in a trial three of more treatments are compared to each other, the typical first statistical analysis is to test the null hypothesis (H_0) of no difference between treatments versus the alternative hypothesis (H_a) that at least one treatment deviates from the others. Suppose that in the trial k different treatments are compared, then the null hypothesis is formulated as $H_0: 3_1 = 3_2 = ... = 3_k$, where 3_i is the treatment-effect of treatment i. When the efficacy variable is quantitative (and normally distributed), then 3 is the mean value. When the efficacy variable is binary (e.g. healthy or ill), then 3 is the proportion of positive (say healthy) patients. When the efficacy variable is of ordinal character, or is a survival time, 3 can have different quantifications. For the remainder of this paragraph we assume that the efficacy is quantitative and normally distributed, because for this situation the multiple comparison procedure has been studied thoroughly.

Consider the randomized clinical trial comparing 5 different treatments for ejaculation praecox[1]: one group of patients received a placebo treatment (group 1), and the four other groups received different serotonin reuptake inhibitors (SSRI). The primary variable for evaluating the efficacy was the logarithmically transformed intravaginal ejaculation latency time (IELT) measured after six weeks of treatment. The null hypothesis in this trial was that there was no difference between the five groups of patients with respect to the mean of the logarithmically transformed IELT: $H_0: 3_1 = 3_2 = 3_3 = 3_4 = 3_5$. The summarizing data of this trial are listed in Table 1.

Table 1. Randomized clinical trial comparing 5 different treatments for ejaculation praecox[1]: one group of patients received a placebo treatment (group 1), and the four other groups received different serotonin reuptake inhibitors (SSRI). The primary variable for evaluating the efficacy was the logarithmically transformed intravaginal ejaculation latency time (IELT) measured after six weeks of treatmen.

Treatment	sample size n	Mean x	Standard deviation S
Placebo	9	3.34	1.14
SSRI A	6	3.96	1.09
SSRI B	7	4.96	1.18
SSRI C	12	5.30	1.51
SSRI D	10	4.70	0.78

The first statistical analysis was done by calculating the analysis of variance (ANOVA) table. The F-test for the testing the null hypothesis had value 4.13 with 4 and 39 degrees of freedom and p-value 0.0070. The within group sums of squares was 55.16 with 39 degrees of freedom, thus the mean squared error was S=1.41. Since the p-value was far below the nominal level of ,=0.05, the null hypothesis could be rejected. This led to the not-too-informative conclusion that not all population averages were equal. A question immediately encountered is which one of the different population did and which one did not differ from each other. This question concerns the problem of multiple comparisons or post-hoc comparison of treatment groups.

The only way of finding out which one of the populations means differ from each other is to compare every treatment group with all of the other groups or with a specified subset receiving other treatments. When there are 5 different treatments, 5x4/2=10 different pairs of treatments can be compared. In general, when there are k treatments, k(k-1)/2 different comparisons can be made.

The easiest approach to this question is to calculate the Student's t-test for each comparison of the groups i and j. This procedure may be refined by using in the denominator of the t-test the pooled-within-group variance S_w^2, as already calculated in the above F-test according to:

$$t_{ij} = \frac{\bar{x}_i - \bar{x}_j}{\sqrt{S_w^2 \left(\frac{1}{n_i} + \frac{1}{n_j} \right)}}. \tag{1}$$

This t-statistic has n-k degrees of freedom, where n is the total number of observations in the entire sample and k is the number of treatment groups. This procedure is called the "least significant difference" procedure (LSD procedure). For the application of the LSD procedure, it is essential to perform it sequentially to a significant F-test of the ANOVA procedure. So if one chooses to perform the LSD procedure, one first calculates the ANOVA procedure and stops if the F-test is non-significant, and calculates the LSD tests only when the F-test is statistically significant. The LSD procedure is largely similar to the Bonferroni-t-test for paired comparisons as explained in Chapter 2 section 3.

When the different treatment groups are compared without performing ANOVA first, or when you do so without the F-test being significant, then the problem of multiple comparisons is encountered. This means that when you make enough comparisons, the chance of finding a significant difference will be substantially larger than the nominal level of ,=0.05: thus the risk of a type-I error will be (far) too large. There may be situations where we want to further the analysis all the same.

There are several ways, then, of dealing with the problem of an increased risk of type-I-error. The easiest method is to use the bonferroni-correction, sometimes known as the modified LSD procedure. The general principle is that the significance level for the experiment, $_{,E}$, is less than or equal to the significance level for each comparison, α_C, times the number of comparisons that are made (remember α is the chance of a type-I-error or the chance of finding a difference where there is none):

$$\alpha_E \leq \frac{k(k-1)}{2} \alpha_C \tag{2}$$

If $_{,E}$ ≤ 0.05, then this level of α is maintained if $_{,C}$ is taken to be , divided by the number of comparisons:

$$\alpha_C = \alpha \frac{2}{k(k-1)}. \tag{3}$$

When k is not too large, this method performs well. However, if k is large (k>5), then the bonferroni correction is overconservative, meaning that the nominal significance level soon will be much lower than ,=0.05 and loss of power occurs accordingly.

There are several alternative methods[2], but here we will discuss briefly three of them: Tukey's honestly significant difference (HSD) method, the Student-Newman-Keuls method, and the method of Dunnett. Tukey's HSD method calculates the test-statistic from the above equation (1), but determines the significance level slightly differently, by considering the distribution of the largest standardized difference $|x_i-x_j|/se(x_i-x_j)$. This distribution is somewhat more complex than that of the t-distribution or of the LSD procedure. A table of significance levels is available in all major statistical books as well as statistical software packages such as SAS and SPSS.[3,4] The HSD procedure controls the maximum experimentwise error rate, and performs well in simulation studies, especially when sample sizes are unequal.

The Student-Newman-Keuls (SNK) procedure is a so-called multiple-stage or multiple range test. The procedure first tests the homogeneity of all k means at the nominal level $_{,k}$. When the homogeneity is rejected, then each subset of (k-1) means is tested for homogeneity at the nominal level $_{,k-1}$, and so on. It does so by calculating the studentized statistic in the above equation (1) for all pairs. The distribution of this statistic is again rather complex, and it depends on the degrees of freedom n-k (from ANOVA), on the number of comparisons that are made, and on $_{,k}$. The table of significance levels is likewise available in most statistical packages. The conclusions of the SNK procedure critically depend on the order of the pairwise comparisons being made. The proper procedure is to compare first the largest mean with the smallest, then the largest with the second-smallest, and so on. An important rule is that if no significant difference exists between two means, it should be concluded that no difference exists between any means enclosed by the two, without further need of testing.

There are many multiple range tests[2], mainly differing in their use of the significance level $_{,k}$ and $_{,k-1}$. The Student-Newman-Keuls procedure uses $_{,k}=,=0.05$, and therefore does not control the maximum experimentwise error rate.

Finally, there is a special multiple comparison procedure for comparing all active treatments to a control or placebo group. This is the socalled Dunnett's procedure. For all treatments the studentized statistic of above equation (1) compared to the placebo group is calculated. In case of Dunnett's procedure, this statistic again has a complex distribution (many-one t-statistic) which depends on the number of active treatment groups, the degrees of freedom and a correlation term which depends on the sample sizes in each treatment group. Tables are likewise available in statistical packages. If sample sizes are not equal, it is important to use the harmonic mean of the sample sizes when calculating the significance of the Dunnett's test.

Most of the statistical packages compute common multiple range tests, and provide associated confidence intervals for the difference in means. In our trial comparing 4 SSRIs and placebo in patients with ejaculation praecox, we were interested in all of the possible comparisons between the five treatment groups. Since the ANOVA F-test was statistically significant, we applied the LSD procedure to find out which treatment differed significantly from each other. We found the following results. HSD procedure, the bonferroni correction, and Dunnett's procedure of the same data were applied for control (table 2).

Table 2. In the trial from Table 1 the investigators were interested in all of the possible comparisons between the five treatment groups. Since the ANOVA F-test was statistically significant, we applied the LSD procedure to find out which treatment differed significantly from each other. We found the following results. HSD procedure, the bonferroni correction, and Dunnett's procedure of the same data were applied for control.

		Difference		P value		
		Mean (SE)	LSD	HSD	Bonferroni	Dunnett
Placebo vs	A	-0.62 (0.63)	0.33	0.86	0.99	0.73
	B	-1.62 (0.60)	0.01	0.07	0.10	0.035
	C	-1.96 (0.52)	0.001	0.005	0.006	0.002
	D	-1.36 (0.55)	0.017	0.12	0.17	0.058
A vs	B	-1.00 (0.66)	0.14	0.56	0.99	
	C	-1.34 (0.60)	0.03	0.18	0.30	
	D	-0.74 (0.61)	0.24	0.75	0.99	
B vs	C	-0.34 (0.57)	0.56	0.98	0.99	
	D	0.26 (0.59)	0.66	0.99	0.99	
C vs	D	0.60 (0.51)	0.25	0.76	0.99	

SE=standard error.

The mean difference indicates the differences of the means of the groups as shown in table 1. The standard error as calculated from the studentized statistic in the equation (1), and is required in order to construct confidence intervals. The critical values for the construction of such confidence intervals are supplied by appropriate tables for the HSD, and Dunnett's procedure, but are also calculated by most statistical software programs. In our case it is obvious that the LSD procedure provides the smallest p-values, and significant differences between SSRIs B, C and D and placebo results, as well as between A and C results. When using the Bonferroni test or the HSD procedure, only SSRI C is significantly different from placebo. Dunnett's test agrees with the LSD procedure with respect to the differences of the SSRIs compared to placebo, but has no information on the differences between the SSRIs.

There is no general consensus on what post-hoc test to use or when to use it; as the statistical community has not yet reached agreement on this issue. The US Food and Drug Agency suggests in its clinical trial handbook for in house usage to describe in the study protocol the arguments for using a specific method, but refrains from making any preference. We have a light preference for calculating an overall test first such as is done with ANOVA, and subsequently proceed with the LSD test.

Unfortunately, so far multiple comparisons methods have not been developed much for discrete, ordinal and censored data. When dealing with such data, it is best to perform first an overall test by chi-square, kruskal-wallis or logrank methods, and afterwards perform pairwise comparisons with a bonferroni correction.

Whatever method for multiple comparisons, its use or the lack of its use should be discussed in the statistical analysis, and preferably be specified in the analysis plan of the study protocol.

3. PRIMARY AND SECONDARY VARIABLES

Most clinical trials use several, and sometimes many, endpoints to evaluate the treatment efficacy. The use of significance tests separately for each endpoint comparison increases the risk of a type-I error of finding a difference where there is none. The statistical analysis should reflect awareness of this very problem, and in the study protocol the use or non-use of statistical adjustments or their lack must be explained. There are several ways of handling this problem of multiple testing.

I.   The most obvious way is to simply reduce the number of endpoint parameters otherwise called primary outcome variable. Preferably, we should include one primary parameter, usually being the variable that provides the most relevant and convincing evidence of the primary objective of the trial. The trial success is formulated in terms of results demonstrated by this very variable, and prior sample size determination is also based on this variable. Other endpoint variables are placed on a lower level of importance and are defined secondary variables. The secondary variable results may be used to support the evidence provided by the primary variable.

It may sometimes be desirable to use two or more primary variables, each of which sufficiently important for display in the primary analysis. The statistical analysis of such an approach should be carefully spelled in the protocol. In particular, it should be stated in advance what result of any of these variables is least required for the purpose of meeting the trial objectives. Of course, if the purpose of the trial is to demonstrate a significant effect in two or more variables, then there is no need for adjustment of the type-I error risk, but the consequence is that the trial fails in its objectives if one of these variables do not produce a significant result. Obviously, such a rule enhances the chance of erroneously negative trials, in a way similar to the risk of negative trials due to small sample sizes.

II   A different more philosophical approach to the problem of multiple outcome variables is to look for trends without judging one or two low P-values among otherwise high P-values as proof. This requires discipline and is particularly efficient when multiple measurements are performed for the purpose of answering one single question, e.g., the benefit to health of a new drug estimated in terms of effect on mortality in addition to a number of morbidity variables. There is nothing wrong with this practice. We should not make any formal correction for multiple comparisons of this kind (see also Chapter 1, section 1). Instead, we should informally integrate all the data before reaching a conclusion.

III   An alternative way of dealing with the multiple comparison problem when there are many primary variables, is to apply a Bonferroni correction. This means that *the p-value of every variable is multiplied by the number of endpoints k.* This ensures that if treatments were truly equivalent, the trial as a whole will have less than a 5% chance of getting any p-value less than 0.05; thus the overall type-I error rate will be less than 5%.

IV   The Bonferroni correction, however, is not entirely correct when multiple comparisons are dependent of each other(multiple comparions in one subject cannot be considered independent of each other, compare chapter 2, section 3, for additional discussion of this issue). Also the Bonferroni correction is an overcorrection in case of larger numbers of endpoints, particularly when different endpoints are (highly) correlated. A somewhat more adequate variation of the Bonferroni correction, was suggested by Hochberg.[5] *When there are k primary values, the idea is to multiply the largest p-value with 1, the second-largest p-value with 2, the third largest p-value with 3, ..., and the smallest p-value with k.* We do not attempt to explain the mathematical arguments of this procedure, but conclude that lowest and highest –values will be less different from each other. In practice, Hochberg's procedure is frequently hardly less conservative than is the Bonferroni correction.

V   An further alternative for analyzing two or more primary variables is to design a summary measure or composite variable. With such an approach endpoint and primary variables must, of course, be assessed in advance, , and the algorithm to calculate the composite must also be specified a priori. Since in this case primary variables are reduced to one composite, there is no need to make adjustments to salvage the type-I error rate. For the purpose of appropriate composite variables there are a few sensible rules to bear in mind:

- Highly correlated variables, measuring more or less the same patient characteristic can best be replaced by their average. In this way the number of primary variables is reduced, and an additional advantage is that the mean is more reliable than both single measurements.
- When the variables have different scales (e.g. blood pressure is measured in mm Hg units, and cholesterol in mmol/L units), the composite variables are best calculated as socalled standardized variables. This means that the overall mean is subtracted from each measurement and that the resulting difference is divided by the overall standard deviation. In this way all variables will have zero mean and unit standard deviation in the total sample.

Well-known examples of composite variables are rating scales routinely used for the assessment of health-related quality of life, as well as disease-activity-scales (e.g., the disease activity scale of Fuchs for patients with reumatoid arthritis, DAS[6]). The DAS is a composite based on the socalled Ritchie joint pain score, the number of swollen joints, and, in addition, the erythrocyte sedimentation rate:

$$DAS = 0.53938\sqrt{ritchie\ index} + 0.06465(number\ of\ swollen\ joints) +$$

$$0.330\ln(erythocyte\ sedimentation\ rate) + 0.224.$$

For the statistical analysis of a composite variable, standard methods may be used without adjustments. Lauter[7] showed that the statistical test for the composite has 5% type-I error rate. He also showed that such a statistical test is especially sensitive when each endpoint variable has more or less the same individual p-value, but that it has little sensitivity when one endpoint variable is much more significant than others.
We applied these methods to a clinical trial of patients with atherosclerosis comparing two-year placebo versus pravastatin medication.[8] The efficacy of this medication was evaluated by assessing the change of total cholesterol, HDL cholesterol, LDL cholesterol, and triglycerides. The mean changes and standard deviations (mmol/L) are given in Table 3, while also the uncorrected p-values, and the corrected p-values according to Bonferroni and Hochberg are reported.

Table 3.Clinical trial of patients with atherosclerosis comparing two-year placebo versus pravastatin medication.[8] The efficacy of this medication was evaluated by assessing the change of total cholesterol, HDL cholesterol, LDL cholesterol, and triglycerides. The mean changes and standard deviations (mmol/L) are given, while also the uncorrected p-values, and the corrected p-values according to Bonferroni and Hochberg are reported

Change of:	Placebo (n=31)	Pravastatin (n=48)	P^*	$P^\#$	$P^@$
Total cholesterol decrease	-0.07 (0.72)	0.25 (0.73)	0.06	0.24	0.11
HDL cholesterol increase	-0.02 (0.18)	0.04 (0.12)	0.07	0.28	0.11
LDL cholesterol decrease	0.34 (0.60)	0.59 (0.65)	0.09	0.36	0.11
Triglycerides increase	0.03 (0.65)	0.28 (0.68)	0.11	0.44	0.11

* p value of Student's t-test; # bonferroni corrected p-value; @ p-value corrected using Hochberg's methods.

It is obvious that none of the changes are statistically significant using a standard t-test, but it is also clear that all four efficacy variables have a treatment difference that points in the same direction, namely of a positive pravastatin effect. When correcting for multiple testing, the p-values are nowhere near statistical significance. A composite variable of the form $z = $ (total cholesterol + HDL + LDL + triglycerides)/4, where the four lipid measurements are standardized, however, did show statistically significant results: the mean of Z in the placebo group was -0.23 (SD 0.59), and the mean of Z in the pravastatin group was 0.15 (SD 0.56), different $p<0.01$, and so, it is appropriate to conclude that pravastatin significantly reduced the composite variable.

VI   Finally, there are several multivariate methods to perform an overall statistical test for which the type-I error risk equals 5%. Equivalently to the situation comparing many different treatment groups, one might argue that the overall test controls the type-I error, and that subsequently to the overall test, one can perform t-tests and the like without adjustment to explore which variables show significant differences. For comparing two treatment groups on several (normally distributed) variables, one may use Hotelling's T-square, which is the multivariate generalization of the Student's t-test. Other methods to compare different groups of patients on several variables are discriminant analysis, variants of principal components analysis and multinominal logistic regression. The discussion of these methods falls outside the scope of this chapter. It suffices to remark that Hotelling's T-square and the other multivariate methods are readily available through most statistical packages.

4.CONCLUSIONS

Multiple group comparison and multiple variable testing is a very common problem when analyzing clinical trials. There is no consensus within the statistical community on how to cope with these problems. It is therefore essential that awareness of the existence of these problems is reflected in the study protocol and the statistical analysis.

5. REFERENCES

1.   Waldinger MD, Hengeveld MW, Zwinderman AH, Olivier B (1998). Effect of SSRI antidepressants on ejaculation: A double-blind, randomized, placebo-controlled study with fluoxetine, fluvoxamine, paroxetine, and sertraline. Journal of Clinical Psychopharmacology, 18 (4): 274-281.
2.   Multiple comparisons boek, Edition University of Leiden , Neth, 1999.
3.   SAS Statistical Software, 1998.
4.   SPSS Statistical Software, Chicago, IL, 1996.
5.   Hochberg Y. A sharper bonferroni procedure for multiple tests of significance. Biometrika 1988, 75: 800-802.
6.   Fuchs HA. The use of the disease activity score in the analysis of clinical trials in rheumatoid arthritis. J Rheumatol, 1993, 20(11): 1863-6.

7. Lauter J. Exact t and F-tests for analyzing studies with multiple endpoints. Biometrics 1996, 52: 964-970.
8. Jukema JW, Bruschke AV, Van Boven AJ, Zwinderman AH, et al. Effects of lipid lowering by pravastatin on the regression of coronary artery disease in symtomatic men. Circulation 1995; 91: 2528-40.

CHAPTER 8

PRINCIPLES OF LINEAR REGRESSION

1 INTRODUCTION

In the past chapters we discussed different statistical methods to test statistically experimental data from clinical trials. We did not emphasize correlation and regression analysis. The point is that correlation and regression analysis test correlations, rather than causal relationships. Two samples may be strongly correlated e.g., two different diagnostic tests for assessment of the same phenomenon. This does ,however, not mean that one diagnostic test causes the other. In testing the data from clinical trials we are mainly interested in causal relationships. When such assessments were statistically analyzed through correlation analyses mainly, we would probably be less convinced of a causal relationship than we are while using prospective hypothesis testing. So, this is the main reason we so far did not address correlation testing extensively. With epidemiological observational research things are essentially different: data are obtained from the observation of populations or the retrospective observation of patients selected because of a particular condition or illness. Conclusions are limited to the establishment of relationships, causal or not. We currently believe that relationships in medical research between a factor and an outcome can only be proven to be causal when the factor is introduced and subsequently gives rise to the outcome. We are more convinced when such is tested in the form of a controlled clinical trial. A problem with multiple regression and logistic regression analysis as method for analyzing of multiple samples in clinical trials is closely related to this point. There is always an air of uncertainty about such regression data. Interventional trials usually use hypothesis-testing and 95 % CI data to describe and analyze data. They use multiple regression for secondary analyses, thus enhancing the substance of the research, and making the readership more willing to read the report, rather than proving the primary endpoints. Regression analysis may not be so important to randomized clinical trials, it is important to one particular study design, the crossover study, where every patient is given in random order test-treatment and standard treatment (or placebo). Figure 1 gives three hypothesized examples of crossover trials. It can be observed from the plots that in the left and right graph there seems to be a linear relationship between treatment one and two. The strength of relationship is expressed as r (=correlation coefficient) which varies between -1 and +1. The strongest association is given by either -1 or +1 (all data exactly on the line), the weakest association 0 (all data are parallel either to x-axis or to y-axis, or half one direction, half the other). A positive correlation in a crossover study is observed if two drugs from one class are compared. The patients responding well to the first drug are more likely to respond well to the second. In contrast, in crossover studies comparing drugs from different classes a negative correlation may be observed: patients not responding well to one class are more likely to respond well to the other.

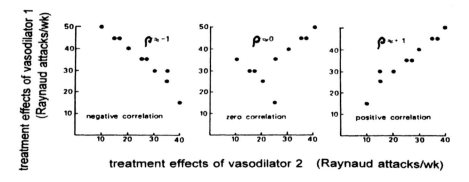

Fig 1. Example of 3 crossover studies of two treatment in patients with Raynaud's phenomenon. the (Pearson's) correlation coefficient r varies between -1 and +1.

2. MORE ON PAIRED OBSERVATIONS

Table 1 gives the real data of a crossover study comparing a new laxant versus a standard laxant, bisacodyl. Days with stool are used as primary endpoint. The table shows that the new drug is more efficaceous than bisacodyl, but the figure shows somethying else: there is a positive correlation between the two treatments: those responding well to bisacodyl are more likely to respond well to the novel laxant.

Table 1. Example of a crossover trial comparing efficacy of a new laxant versus bisacodyl

patient no.	new treatment (y-variables) (days with stool)	bisacodyl (x-variables) (days of stool)
1	24	8
2	30	13
3	25	15
4	35	10
5	39	9
6	30	10
7	27	8
8	14	5
9	39	13
10	42	15
11	41	11
12	38	11
13	39	12
14	37	10
15	47	18
16	30	13
17	36	12
18	12	4
19	26	10
20	20	8
21	43	16
22	31	15
23	40	14
24	31	7
25	36	12
26	21	6
27	44	19
28	11	5
29	27	8
30	24	9
31	40	15
32	32	7
33	10	6
34	37	14
35	19	7

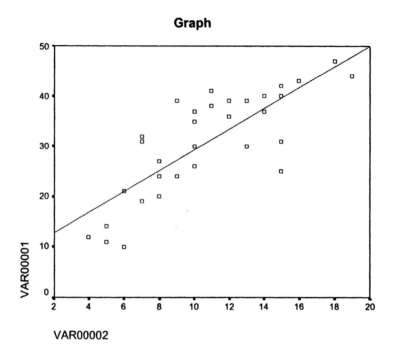

Fig 1. Scatterplot of data from Table 1 with regression line.

A regression line can be calculated from the data according to the equation

$$y=a+bx$$

The line drawn from this linear function provides the best fit for the data given, where y = socalled dependent, and x = independent variable, b = regression coefficient.

a and b from the equation y=a+bx can be calculated.

$$b = \text{regression coefficient} = \sqrt{\frac{\Sigma(x - \bar{x})(y - \bar{y})}{\Sigma(x - \bar{x})^2}}$$

$$a = \text{intercept} = \bar{y} - b\bar{x}$$

r = correlation coefficient = is another important determinant and looks a lot like b.

$$r = \sqrt{\frac{\Sigma(x - \bar{x})(y - \bar{y})}{\Sigma(x - \bar{x})^2 \Sigma(y - \bar{y})^2}}$$

r = measure for the strength of association between y and x-data. The stronger the association, the better y predicts x.

3 USING STATISTICAL SOFTWARE FOR SIMPLE LINEAR REGRESSION

Regression analysis without software is laborious. We may use a computer progam, e.g., **SPSS Statistical Software**, to do the job for us. We command our software: **Statistics; Regression; Linear**.

The software calculates the values b and a and r so as to minimize the sum of the squared vertical distances of the points from the line (socalled least squares fit). **SPSS 8 for windows 99** provides us with three tables: **(1) Model Summary, (2) ANOVA, (3) coefficients**.

Table 2

Model Summary

Model	R	R Square	Adjusted R Square	Std. Error of the Estimate
1	.794[a]	.630	.618	6.1590

a. Predictors: (Constant), VAR00002

ANOVA[b]

Model		Sum of Squares	df	Mean Square	F	Sig.
1	Regression	2128.393	1	2128.393	56.110	.000[a]
	Residual	1251.779	33	37.933		
	Total	3380.171	34			

a. Predictors: (Constant), VAR00002
b. Dependent Variable: VAR00001

Coefficients[a]

Model		Unstandardized Coefficients		Standardized Coefficients	t	Sig.
		B	Std. Error	Beta		
1	(Constant)	8.647	3.132		2.761	.009
	VAR00002	2.065	.276	.794	7.491	.000

a. Dependent Variable: VAR00001

(1) Model Summary gives information on correlation coefficient and its square the socalled coefficient of determination. A coefficient of determination of 0.63 indicates that 63% of the variation in the y variable is explained by variation in the x variable. The better the effect of bisacodyl the better the novel laxant is going to work. Adjusted r square is important for small samples only while std error of the estimate tells us something about the residu (variance not explained by the regression).

At this point it is important to consider the following. Before doing any regression analysis we have to make the assumptions that our data are normally distributed and that variances in x ands y-variable do not show a lot of difference, otherwise called heteroscedasticity (heteroscedasticity literally means "different SDs").

White's Test is a simple method to check for this. Chi-square table is used for that purpose.

if $n r^2 < \chi^2 (n)$ we don't have to worry about heteroscedasticity.

n= sample size

r= correlation coefficient

$\chi^2 (n)$ = the value for n degrees of freedom.

In our example 35 (0.630) = 22.05 while χ^2 (35) = 16.70 (no heteroscedasticity)

(2) ANOVA shows how the paired data can be assessed in the form of analysis of variance. Variations are expressed as sums of squares. The total variation in the regression is divided into sum of squares (SS) regression, or variances explained by the regression, and SS residual, variances unexplained by the regression.

$$r^2 = \frac{(\Sigma(x - \bar{x})(y - \bar{y}))^2}{\Sigma(x - \bar{x})^2 \Sigma(y - \bar{y})^2} = \frac{SP^2 x.y}{SS x \,.\, SS y}$$

where SP = sum of products x . y

SS regression = SP^2 xy / SSx = 2128.393

SS total = SS y

SS regression/ SS total= 2128.393/ SS total = 0.63 (= r square (Model Summary))

The F-test is helpful to reject the null-hypothesis that r=0. We reject this null-hypothesis at a p<0.00. There is thus a significant correlation between the y and x variables.

(3) Coefficients shows the real regression equation. The intercept is named "(constant)" and given under B = 8.647. The b-value in the linear regression equation is 2.065.

The regression equation is thus as follows.

y= 8.647 + 2.065 . x

new laxant= 8.647 + 2.065 . bisacodyl

In addition to unstandardized coefficients, standardized coefficients are given. For that purpose SSy is defined to be 1. Then, r = b. Instead of testing the null-hypothesis that r = 0, we can now test that b=0, and use for that purpose the t-test. The t-value of 7.491 = $\sqrt{F}$= $\sqrt{56.110}$ (from the ANOVA Table).

4 MULTIPLE LINEAR REGRESSION

We may be interested to know if age is an independent contributor to the effect of the new laxant. For that purpose a simple regression equation has to be extended as follows

y= a + $b_1 x_1$ + $b_2 x_2$

b_i are called partial regression coefficients. Just like simple linear regression, multiple linear regression can give us the best fit for the data given, although it is hard to display the correlations in a figure. Table 2 gives the data from Table 1 extended by the variable age. <

Table 3. Example of a crossover trial comparing efficacy of a new laxant versus bisacodyl

patient no.	new treatment y-variables (days with stool)	bisacodyl x_1 -variables (days with stool)	age x_2 -variables (years)
1	24	8	25
2	30	13	30
3	25	15	25
4	35	10	31
5	39	9	36
6	30	10	33
7	27	8	22
8	14	5	18
9	39	13	14
10	42	15	30
11	41	11	36
12	38	11	30
13	39	12	27
14	37	10	38
15	47	18	40
16	30	13	31
17	36	12	25
18	12	4	24
19	26	10	27
20	20	8	20
21	43	16	35
22	31	15	29
23	40	14	32
24	31	7	30
25	36	12	40
26	21	6	31
27	44	19	41
28	11	5	26
29	27	8	24
30	24	9	30
31	40	15	20
32	32	7	31
33	10	6	29
34	37	14	43
35	19	7	30

The table 3 shows too many data to allow any conclusions. We use for assessment of these data the same SPSS program called linear regression and command again: **Statistics; Regression; Linear.** The software **SPSS 8 for windows 99** provides us with the following three subtables: **(1) Model Summary, (2) ANOVA, (3) coefficients.**

Table 4

Model Summary

Model	R	R Square	Adjusted R Square	Std. Error of the Estimate
1	.848[a]	.719	.701	5.4498

a. Predictors: (Constant), VAR00003, VAR00002

ANOVA[b]

Model		Sum of Squares	df	Mean Square	F	Sig.
1	Regression	2429.764	2	1214.882	40.905	.000[a]
	Residual	950.407	32	29.700		
	Total	3380.171	34			

a. Predictors: (Constant), VAR00003, VAR00002
b. Dependent Variable: VAR00001

Coefficients[a]

Model		Unstandardized Coefficients		Standardized Coefficients	t	Sig.
		B	Std. Error	Beta		
1	(Constant)	-1.547	4.233		-.366	.717
	VAR00002	1.701	.269	.653	6.312	.000
	VAR00003	.426	.134	.330	3.185	.003

a. Dependent Variable: VAR00001

(1)Model Summary shows r, here called the multiple r, The corresponding "multiple r square", otherwise called coefficient of determination, of 0.719 indicates that 71.9 % of the variation in the y variable is explained by variation in the two x variables. Interestingly, the multiple r square is a bit larger than the simple r square (0.719 and 0.618). Information is thus given about the perfection of the model. After the first step 61.8 % of variation is explained by the regression model, after the second no less than 71.9% is explained by it. The addition of age to the model produces 71.9-63= 8.9% extra explanation of the variance in the y variable, the effect of the new laxant.

Before going further we have to consider the hazard of collinearity, which is the situation where two x variables are highly correlated. One naive though common way in which collinearity is introduced into the data, is through inclusion of x variables that are actually the same measures under different names. This is, obviously, not so with bisacodyl effect and age. Nonetheless, we measure the presence of collinearity by calculating the simple correlation coeffcient between the x variables before doing anything more. In our case r between x_1 variables and x_2 variables is 0.425, and so we don't have to worry about (multi)collinearity (r>0.90).

(2)**ANOVA** can test the null hypothesis that r=0. Again SS regression (by regression explained variance) is divided by SS residual (unexplained variance), the total variance being SS regression + SS residual. The division sum 304.570/ SS total yields 0.719 = r square.

(3)**Coefficients** again shows the real regression equation. The intercept a is given by the (constant). The b values are the unstandardized regression coefficients of the x_1 and x_2 variables.

The regression equation is thus as follows

$y = -1.547 + 1.701 . x_1 + 0.426 . x_2$

new laxant $= -1.547 + 1.701 .$ bisacodyl $+ 0.426 .$ age

In addition to unstandardized coefficients, standardized coefficients are given. For that purpose SS y is taken to be 1. Then r = b. Instead of testing the null hypothesis that r= 0 we can now test that various b_i = 0, and use for that purpose t-test. As both bisacodyl and age are significantly correlated with the y variable(the efficacy of the new laxant), both x variables are independent predictors of the efficacy of the new laxant.

5 ANOTHER REAL DATA EXAMPLE OF MULTIPLE LINEAR REGRESSION

We want to study "Independent determinants of quality of life of patients with angina pectoris". Note this is an observational rather than interventional study. We give the example because these kinds of data are often obtained as secondary data from interventional studies.

y-variable= index of quality of life of patients with stable angina pectoris
x-variables=1.Age
        2.Gender
        3.Rhythm disturbances
        4.Peripheral vascular disease
        5.Concomitant calcium channel blockers
        6.Concomitant beta blockers
        7.NYHA-classification
        8.Smoking
        9.body mass index
        10.hypercholesterolemia
        11.hypertension
        12.diabetes mellitus

Index of quality of life $= a + b_1 (age) + 1b_2 (gender) + \ldots\ldots b_{12} (diabetes)$

Correlation between independent variables may be correlated but not too closely: e.g. body mass index, body weight, body length should not be included all three. We used single linear regression for assessing this correlation, otherwise called multicollinearity.

Table 5 correlation matrix in order to test multicollinearity in the regression analysis, P-values are given

	age	gender	rhythm	vasc dis	ccb	bb	NYHA	smoking	bmi	chol	hypt
gender	0.19										
rhythm	0.12	ns									
vasc dis	0.14	ns	ns								
ccb	0.24	ns	0.07	ns							
bb	0.33	ns	ns	ns	0.07						
NYHA	0.22	ns	ns	0.07	0.07	ns					
smoking	–0.12	ns	0.09	0.07	0.08	ns					
bmi	0.13	ns	ns	ns	ns	0.10	-0.07				
chol	0.15	ns	ns	0.12	0.09	ns	0.08	0.09			
hypt	0.09	ns	0.08	ns	0.10	0.09	0.09	0.09	0.07		
diabetes	0.12	ns	0.09	0.10	ns	0.08	ns	0.11	0.12	0.10	

vasc dis= peripheral vascular disease; ccb= calcium channel blocker therapy; bb= beta-blocker therapy; bmi= body mass index; hypt= hypertension; ns= not statistically significantly correlated (Pearson correlation P-value>0.05)

Table 6 Regression Coëfficients and Standard Errors for a Multiple Linear Regression of the index of quality-of-life-during-optimized-nitrate-therapy on various concomitant variables (=covariates)

Covariate level	estimated regression coëfficient	estimated standard error	test statistic (T)	Significance (P-value)
Age	-0.03	0.04	0.8	0.39
Gender	001	0.05	0.5	0.72
Rhythm disturbances	-0.04	0.04	1.0	0.28
Peripheral vascular disease	-0.00	0.01	0.1	0.97
Calcium channel blockers	0.00	0.01	0.1	0.99
beta blockers	0.03	0.04	0.7	0.43
NYHA-classification	-0.08	0.03	2.3	0.02
Smoking	-0.06	0.04	1.6	0.08
body mass index	-0.07	0.03	2.1	0.04
hypercholesterolemia	0.07	0.03	2.2	0.03
hypertension	-0.08	0.03	2.3	0.02
diabetes mellitus	0.06	0.03	2.0	0.05

NYHA= New York Heart Association

Conclusions: The higher the NYHA class the lower quality of life. Smokers , obese subjects, and patients with concomitant hypertension have lower quality of life. Patients with cholesterolemia or diabetes mellitus have better quality of life. The latter two categories have early endothelial dysfunction and may have significant angina pectoris with fairly intact coronary arteries.

6 CONCLUSIONS

If you are frustrated now, don´t be: multiple linear regression analyis and its extensions like logistic regression and Cox´s proportional hazard model is not as important for clinical trials as it is for observational research:
1. Regression analysis assesses associations not causalities.
2. Clinical trials assess causal relationships.
3. We believe in causality if factor is introduced and gives rise to a particular outcome.
4. Always air of uncertainty with regression analysis

Multiple linear regression is interesting, but, in the context of clinical trials mostly just exploratory.

CHAPTER 9

SUBGROUP ANALYSIS USING MULTIPLE LINEAR REGRESSION: CONFOUNDING, INTERACTION, SYNERGISM

1. INTRODUCTION

When the size of the study permits, important demographic or baseline value-defined subgroups of patients can be studied for unusually large or small efficacy responses; e.g. comparison of effects by age, sex; by severity or prognostic groups. Naturally, such analyses are not intended to "salvage" an otherwise negative study, but may be may be helpful in refining patient or dose selection for subsequent studies.[1]

Most studies have insufficient size to assess efficacy meaningfully in subgroups of patients. Instead a regression model for the primary or secondary efficacy-variables can be used to evaluate whether specific variables are confounders for the treatment effect, and whether the treatment effect interacts with specific covariates. The particular (statistical) regression model chosen, depends on the nature of the efficacy variables, and the covariates to be considered should be meaningful according to the current state of knowledge. In particular, when studying interactions, the results of the regression analysis are more valid when complemented by additional exploratory analyses within relevant subgroups of patients or within strata defined by the covariates.

In this chapter we will discuss the multiple linear regression model which is appropriate, for continuous efficacy variables, such as blood pressure or lipid level (as discussed in chapter 2). Regression models for dichotomous efficacy variables (logistic regression[2]), and for survival data (Cox regression[3]) will not be assessed here. However, the principles underlying all of these models are to some extent equivalent.

2. EXAMPLE

As an example of the use of a regression model we consider trials such as those conducted to evaluate the efficacy of statins (HMG-CoA reductase inhibitors) to lower lipid levels in patients with atherosclerosis[4]. In unselected populations statins were extremely effective in lowering LDL-cholesterol (LDL), but the question whether the efficacy depended on baseline LDL level was unanswered. Of course this could be asnwered by comparing efficacy in selected subgroups of patients with baseline *low*, *intermediate*, and *high* LDL levels, but a regression model could be used as well, and sometimes provides better sensitivity.

Consider a randomized clinical trial such as Regress[4]. In this trial 884 patients with documented coronary atherosclerosis and total cholesterol in between 4 and 8 mmol/L were randomized to either two-year pravastatin or placebo treatment. Efficacy of treatment was assessed by the fall in LDL cholesterol after two year treatment. In the n_1=438 patients who received pravastatin mean LDL chlesterol fell by $\bar{x}_1$=1.2324 mmol/L (standard deviation, S_1=0.68). In the n_0=422 available patients who received placebo, the mean LDL cholesterol fell by $\bar{x}_0$=-0.0376 mmol/L (S_0=0.589). Consequently, the efficacy of pravastatin was 1.2324- -0.0376 = 1.2700 mmol/L LDL-decrease in two years with standard error (SE) 0.043, and the 95% confidence interval (ci) of the efficacy quantification ran from 1.185 to 1.355.

In a random patient with coronary atherosclerosis and total cholesterol in between 4 and 8 mmol/L, pravastatin produces a better reduction in LDL cholesterol than does placebo by 1.27 mmol/L. However, a patient with 8 mmol/L total cholesterol level may better benefit than a patient with 4 mmol/L at baseline may do. Multiple linear regression can be applied to assess this question..

3. MODEL(FIGURE 1)

We first introduce some notation: the dependent variable Y_i is the amount of LDL decrease observed in patient i (i=1,...,884), and the independent variable or covariate X_{1i} is an indicator variable, indicating whether patient i received pravastatin (X_{1i}=1) or not (X_{1i}=0). We define the linear regression model:

$$Y_i = \beta_0 + \beta_1 X_{1i} + e_i,$$

where β_0 is the intercept, and β_1 the slope of the regression line and e_i is a residual variation term, which is assumed to be normally distributed with variance σ_e^2.

When X_{1i} is either zero or one, the usual estimates b_0, b_1, and S_e^2 of β_0, β_1, and Σ_e^2 are:

$$b_0 = \bar{x}_0 = -0.0376, \quad b_1 = \bar{x}_1 - \bar{x}_0 = 1.2700, \text{ and}$$

$$S_e^2 = \frac{(n_1 - 1)S_1^2 + (n_0 - 1)S_0^2}{n_1 + n_0 - 2} = 0.4058,$$

which are exactly the same statistics as used in the t-test procedure one would normally employ in this situation. The quantification of the efficacy is thus given by b_1 and it has the same value and the same standard error and confidence interval as above. In figure 1 the linear regression line is illustrated.

Note: b and s are the best estimates, otherwise called best fits, of β and Σ

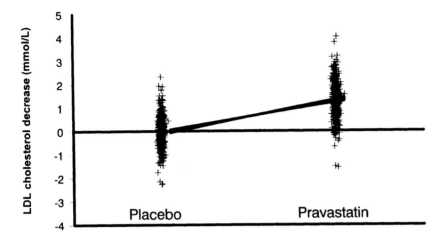

Figure 1. The linear regression line is illustrated.

By using this regression model the following assumptions are made.

1. The relation between Y and X is linear. When X can attain only two values, this assumption is naturally valid, but this is not necessarily so.
2. The distribution of the residual term e_i is normal with mean zero and variance Σ_e^2.
3. The variance of the distribution of e (Σ_e^2) is the same for $X_1=0$ and for $X_1=1$: homoscedasticity.
4. The residual term e_i is independent of X_{1i}.

The object of regression modeling in clinical trials is to evaluate whether the efficacy quantification b_1 (I.) can be made more precise by taking covariates into consideration, (II.) is confounded by covariates, and (III.) interacts with covariates (synergism).
Increased precision (I.) is attained, and confounding (II.) can be studied by extending the regression model with a second independent variable X_2:

$$Y_i = \beta_0 + \beta_1 X_{1i} + \beta_2 X_{2i} + e_i.$$

This multiple regression model has the same underlying assumptions as the above linear regression model (1) except for the assumption that e_i is independent not only of X_1 but also of X_2. There is no need to assume that X_1 and X_2 are strictly independent, but the association must not be too strong (multicollinearity).

4. (I.) INCREASED PRECISION OF EFFICACY(FIGURE 2)

When X_2 is independent of X_1 and is associated with Y (thus $b_2 \neq 0$), the estimate b_1 of the model in equation (2) will be the same as the estimate b_1 of the model in equation (1), but its precision will be increased, as indicated by a smaller standard error.

This is a common case in randomized clinical trials. The randomization will ensure that no inbalancies exist between the two treatment groups with respect to covariates such as X_2, and consequently X_2 will be independent of the treatment variable X_1. There are often many candidates for inclusion as covariates in the multiple regression model, but the choice should be made a priori and specified in the protocol. When the dependent variable is a change score, as in our example, the baseline level is the first candidate to consider because it is almost surely associated with the change score Y. Figure 2 shows the relationship between result of treatment and baseline values as demonstrated by scatterplots and linear regression lines for each treatment separately. The multiple linear regression model in equation (2) is appropriate for testing the contribution of baseline variability to the overall variability in the data.

Since X_2 is independent of X_1, inclusion of X_2 in the model must lead to a decreased variance S_e^2: some differences between patients with respect to the LDL decrease, are attributed to baseline LDL levels. Thus there will be less residual variation. Since the standard error of b_1 is a monotonic positive function of S_e^2, a decrease of S_e^2 leads to a smaller standard error of b_1. Thus by including baseline LDL levels in the regression model, the efficacy of pravastatin lowering is estimated more precisely. This rule, however, only applies to large data-sets. With every additional covariate in the model an extra regression weight must be estimated, and since S_e^2 is an inverse function of the number of covariates in the model, too many covariates in the model will lead to decreased precision.

In our example the mean baseline LDL levels (X_2) were 4.32 (SD 0.78) and 4.29 (SD 0.78) in the placebo and pravastatin treatment groups (X_1) (p=0.60); hence X_1 and X_2 were independent. The baseline LDL levels were, however, associated with the LDL-changes (Y): b_2=0.41 (SE 0.024), p<0.0001. Consequently, the estimated efficacy was (almost) the same as before, but it had smaller standard error:

with baseline LDL cholesterol levels: $b_1 = 1.27$ (SE 0.037)
without baseline LDL cholesterol levels: $b_1 = 1.27$ (SE 0.043)

It is important to emphasize that in the extended multiple regression model, the efficacy of pravastatin to lower LDL is, still, independent of baseline LDL cholesterol level:

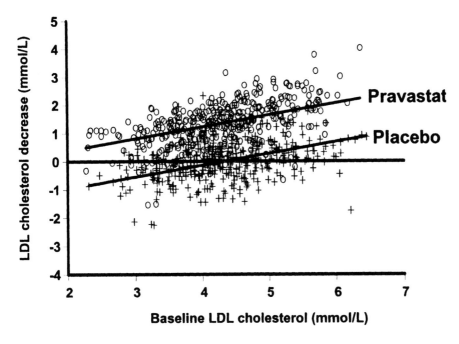

Figure 2. Scatterplots and linear regression lines of baseline LDL cholesterol and LDL cholesterol decrease after treatment, separately for placebo and for pravastatin treatments.

Nota bene: in contrast to the linear regression models the efficacy estimates of non-linear regression models (e.g. logistic[2] and Cox regression[3]) do <u>not</u> remain the same in this case. When using logistic or Cox regression it is therefore imperative to report the log odds ratio or log hazard ratio of treatments compared, together with the covariates in the model.

5. (II.) CONFOUNDING

In randomized clinical trials confounding plays a minor role in the data. The randomization will ensure that no covariate of the efficacy variable will also be associated with the randomized treatment. When, however, the randomization fails for a particular variable, which is already known to be an important covariate of the efficacy variable, such variable is a confounder and adjustment of the efficacy estimate should be attempted. This is done by using the same (linear) regression model as given in equation (2). The adjusted efficacy estimate may become smaller or larger than the unadjusted estimate, depending on the direction of the associations of the confounder with the randomized treatment and the efficacy variable. Let b_1 and $b_1^{\bullet}$ denote the unadjusted and the adjusted efficacy estimate, and let r_{xz} and r_{yz} be the correlations of the confounder (z) with the randomized treatment (x) and the efficacy variable (y), then the following will hold:

$$\text{if} \quad r_{xz}>0 \text{ and } r_{yz}>0 \quad \text{then} \quad |b_1^*|<|b_1|,$$

$$\text{if} \quad r_{xz}>0 \text{ and } r_{yz}<0 \quad \text{then} \quad |b_1^*|>|b_1|,$$

$$\text{if} \quad r_{xz}>0 \text{ and } r_{yz}<0 \quad \text{then} \quad |b_1^*|>|b_1|,$$

$$\text{if} \quad r_{xz}>0 \text{ and } r_{yz}<0 \quad \text{then} \quad |b_1^*|>|b_1|,$$

Notice the possibility that the unadjusted efficacy estimate b_1 is zero whereas the adjusted estimate b_1^* is unequal to zero: an efficacy-difference between treatments may be masked by confounding.

In clinical trials it is sensible to check the balance between treatment groups of all known covariates of the efficacy variable. In most trials there are many more covariates and one should be careful to consider as a confounder a covariate which was not reported in the literature before.

6. (III.) INTERACTION AND SYNERGISM

A special kind of covariate is the interaction of the randomized treatment with some other covariate. This interaction is, by definition, associated with the randomized treatment, and possibly with the efficacy variable if the efficacy differs between treatments. In contrast to the discussion above, the focus of the statistical analysis is not on the change of b_1 by including an interaction in the model, but the regression weight of the interaction variable itself. When this regression weight is unequal to zero, this points to the existence of patient-subgroups for which the efficacy of treatment differs significantly.

An example is again provided by the Regress trial[4]. The primary effect variable was the decrease of the average diameter of the coronary arteries after two years of treatment. The average decrease was 0.057 mm (SD 0.194) in the pravastatin group, and it was 0.117 mm (SD 0.212) in the placebo group (t-test: $p<0.001$); thus the efficacy estimate b_1 was 0.060 (standard error SE=0.016). Calcium channel blockers (CCB) were given to 60% of the placebo patients, and 59% of the pravastatin patients (chi-square: p=0.84): thus CCB treatment was not a confounder variable. Also, CCB medication was not associated with diameter decrease (p=0.62). In the patients who did not receive concomitant CCB medication, the diameter decreases were 0.097 (SD 0.20) and 0.088 (SD 0.19) in patients receiving placebo and pravastatin, respectively (p=0.71). In patients who did receive CCB medication, the diameter decreases were 0.130 (SD 0.22) and 0.035 (SD 0.19), respectively (p<0.001). Thus, pravastatin-efficacy was, on average, 0.097-0.088=0.009 mm in patients without CCB medication, and 0.130-0.035=0.095 in patients with CCB medication.

This difference was statistically significant (interaction test: p=0.011). We used the following linear regression model for this test. Let $X_{1i}=1$ denote that patient i received pravastatin ($X_{1i}=0$, if not), let $X_{2i}=1$ denote that patient i received CCB medication ($X_{2i} = 0$, if not), and let $X_{3i}=X_{1i}*X_{2i}$:

$$Y_i = \beta_0 + \beta_1 X_{1i} + \beta_2 X_{2i} + \beta_3 X_{3i} + e_i.$$

The estimates were: $b_3=0.085$ (SE 0.033), $b_2=-0.033$ (SE 0.023), and $b_1=0.009$ (SE 0.026). Notice that b_1 changed dramatically by including the interaction term X_3 in the linear model; this is a general feature of regression models with interaction terms: the corresponding main-effects (b_1 and b_2) cannot be interpreted independently of the interaction term. Another consequence is that the efficacy estimate no longer exists, but several estimates do exist: in our case there are different efficacy-estimates for patients with ($b_1+b_3=0.009+0.085=0.094$) and without CCB medication ($b_1=0.009$).

In the practice of clinical trials interactions are usually investigated in an exploratory fashion. When interaction is demonstrated in this way, its existence should be confirmed in a novel prospective clinical trial.

7. ESTIMATION, AND HYPOTHESIS TESTING

Standard statistical computer programs like SPSS and SAS (and many others) contain modules that perform regression analysis for linear and many non-linear models such as logistic and Cox regression. The standard method to estimate the linear regression weights (and the residual standard deviation Σ_e) is to minimize the squared distances between the data and the estimated regression line: the least squares method. For non-linear models, the maximum likelihood method is employed, but these are equivalent methods. The output of these estimation methods are the estimated regression weights (and the residual standard deviation Σ_e) and their standard errors. It is important that the correlations between the covariates in the model are not too large (i.e. multicollinearity), but if these are too large this will become clear by absurd regression weights, and very large standard errors. If this occurs one or more covariates must be removed from the model.

Under the null hypothesis that β equals zero, the ratio of the estimated regression weight b and its standard error is distributed as a student's t statistic in the linear model, and this can be used to derive the p-value or the 95% confidence interval in the usual way. For non-linear models, the squared ratio of b and its standard error is called the Wald statistic which is chi-squared distributed. Alternatives for the Wald statistic are the score and likelihood ratio statistics[5], but these give the same results except in highly unusual circumstances; when they differ the score and likelihood statistics are better than the Wald statistic.

The power of these statistical tests is a sensitive function of the number of patients in the trial. Naturally, there is less opportunity for modeling in a small trial than in a large trial. There is no general rule about which sample sizes are required for sensible regression modeling, but one rule-of-thumb is that at least ten times as many patients are required as the number of covariates in the model.

8. GOODNESS-OF-FIT

For the linear model the central assumptions are (1.) the assumed linearity of the relation between Y and X, and (2.) the normal distribution of the residual term e independent of all covariates and with homogeneous variance. The first step in checking these assumptions is by looking at the data. The linearity of the relation between Y and X, for instance, can be inspected by looking at the scatter-plot between Y and X. A nonlinear relation between Y and X will show itself as systematic deviation from a straight line. When the relation is nonlinear, either Y or X or both may be transformed appropriately; most often used are the logarithmic transformation $X^*=\ln(X)$ and the power transformation $X^*=X^p$ (e.g. the squared root transformation where $p=0.5$). At this stage subjective judgments necessarily enter the statistical analysis, because the decision about the appropriate transformation is not well founded on statistical arguments. A few tools that may help, are the following.

1. The optimal power-transformation (X^p) may be estimated using the Box-Cox algorithm[6]. This may yield, however, difficult and unpractical power-transforms.

2. A 'better' model has higher multiple correlation. When one compares two different transformations, the best transformation leads to a smaller residual variance (S_e^2) or higher multiple correlation (R): $S_e^2 =((n-1)/(n-k))(1-R^2)S_y^2$, and (k-1) is the number of covariates in the model.

3. Choosing an appropriate transformation may be avoided by modeling the relation between Y and X as a polynomial function of X: $Y=b_0+b_1X+b_2X^2+b_3X^3+....$. When the relation is strictly linear then $b_2=b_3=...=0$, and this can be tested statistically in the usual way. Obviously, the order of the polynomial function is unknown, but one rarely needs to investigate fourth or higher orders.

4. Finally, there exists the possibility to model the association between Y and X nonparametrically using various modern smoothing techniques.

The assumed normal distribution of the residual term can be checked by inspecting the histogram of e. The estimation method and the hypothesis testing is quite robust against skewed distributions of the residual term, but it is sensible to check for extreme skewness and the occurrence of important outlying data-points. Visual inspection is usually sufficient but one may check the distribution statistically with the Kolmogorov-Smirnov test.

More important is the assumption of homogeneity of the residual variance S: this entails that the variation of e is more or less the same for all values of X. One may check this visually by inspecting the scatterplot of e (or Y) versus X. When heterogeneity is present, again an appropriate transformation of Y may help. If the ratio of S_e/y is equal for various levels of X, the logarithmic transformation $Y^*=\ln(Y)$

may help, and when S_e^2/y^2 is equal for various levels of X, the square-root transformation is appropriate: $Y^* = (Y)^{0.5}$. The independence of the residual term e of all covariates X in the model can be tested with the Durbin-Watson test.

In the logistic regression model the most important underlying assumption is the assumed logistic form of the function linking the covariates to the binary efficacy variable. When not all relevant covariates are in the model, it can be shown that the link-function is not logistic. One way to test this statistically, is by using the Hosmer-Lemeshow test[2]. But when the logistic regression model does not fit, this is of little consequence because this usually points to missing covariates, and these are often not available. In Cox regression, the cardinal underlying assumption is the assumed proportionality of the hazard rates. There are several statistical tests for this assumption; when proportionality does not hold, accelerated failure time models can be used, or the time axis may be partitioned into several periods in which proportionality does hold.

9. SELECTION PROCEDURES

In clinical trials usually many variables are sampled, and often many of these are candidates for inclusion in the regression model. A major problem is the selection of a subset of variables to include in the regression model. By far preferable is to select a (small) set of candidate variables on clinical and theoretical grounds, but if that is not possible a few rules are helpful in the selection process.

1. If the number of covariates is not too large, it is best not to use any selection at all, but simply include all candidates in the regression model. Often it is necessary to shrink the regression weights, using, for instance, a penalty function.

2. When the number of covariates is very large, backward selection methods are preferable to forward selection models. This is usually done according to the p-value or the size of the test-statistic-value.

3. Since the overriding interest of the regression modelling is the estimation of the efficacy of the randomized treatments, the safest course is to be liberal about including covariates in the model: use a p-value of 0.10 or even 0.20 to include covariates in the model.

10. CONCLUSION

The regular statistical analysis of the data of clinical trials should be extended by (exploratory) analysis if the existence of subgroups of patients for which the efficacy estimate differs, is suspected. An efficient way of doing this is by the use of regression analysis. When such subgroups are identified, the exploratory nature of the regression analysis should be emphasized and the subgroup issue should be further assessed in subsequent independent and prospective data-sets.

11. REFERENCES

1. Department of Health and Human Services, Food and Drug Administration. International Conference on Harmonisation; Guidance on Statistical Principles for Clinical Trials Availability. Federal Register, 63 (179), 1998: 49583-49598.
2. Hosmer DW, Lemeshow S. Applied Logistic Regression. New York: Wiley, 1989.
3. Boek over Cox.
4. Jukema AJ, Zwinderman AH, et al for the REGRESS study group. Effects of lipid lowering by pravastatin on progression and regression of coronary artery disease in symptomatic men with normal to moderately elevated serum cholesterol levels. The Regression Growth Evaluation Statin Study (REGRESS). Circulation. 1995 May 15; 91(10): 2528-40
5. Rao CR. Linear Statistical Inference and Its Applications. New York: Wiley, 1973.
6. Box Cox, Statistical Software, University Leiden, Netherlands, 1999.

CHAPTER 10

CURVILINEAR REGRESSION

1. SUMMARY

Figure 1 upper graph shows a plot of data suggesting a curvilinear rather than linear relationship between the x- and y-values. Polynomial regression analysis or Fourier analysis can be used to study these data. Polynomial analysis is an extension of simple linear regression, where a model is used to allow for the existence of other kinds of systematic dependence of the independent y variable (blood presure) on the dependent x variable (time).

Extension from the basic model can be done as follows:

$y = a + bx$	(first order) linear relationship
$y = a + bx + cx^2$	(second order) parabolic relationship
$y = a + bx + cx^2 + dx^3$	(third order) hyperbolic relationship
$y = a + bx + cx^2 + dx^3 + ex^4$	(fourth order) sinusoidal relationship

where a is the intercept and b, c, d, and e are the partial regression coefficients. Statistical software can be used to calculate for the data the regression line that best minimizes the sums of the squared vertical distances of the points from the line and thus provides the best fit for the data. In addition, regression lines of higher than 4 orders can be calculated.

Fourier analysis is the traditional way of analyzing these type of data, and is given by the function

$$f(x) = p + q_1 \cos(x) + .. + q_n \cos n(x) + r_1 \sin(x) + .. + r_n \sin n(x)$$

with p, $q_1...q_n$, and $r_1...r_n$ = constants for the best fit of the given data.

2. AN EXAMPLE: CURVILINEAR REGRESSION ANALYSIS OF AMBULATORY BLOOD PRESSURE MEASUREMENTS

Ambulatory blood pressure monitoring (ABPM) using light weight automated portable equipment has greatly contributed to our understanding of the circadian patterns of blood pressures in individual patients[1] as well as to the study of effects of antihypertensive drugs in groups of patients.[2] However, a problem is that ABPM data using mean values of arbitrarily separated day – and nighttime hours are poorly reproducible[3,4], undermining the validity of this diagnostic tool. Previous studies have demonstrated that both in normo-[5] and in hypertensive groups[6] time is a more powerful source of variation in 24 hour ABPM data than were other sources of variation (between P<0.01 and <0.001 versus between N.S. and <0.01). This reflects the importance of the circadian rhythm in the interpretation of ABPM data, and the need for an assessment that accounts for this very rhythm more adequately than does the means of separated day- and nighttime hours. We also demonstrated that polynomial curves can be produced of ABPM data from both normo-[5] and hypertensive[6] groups, and that these polynomial curves are within the 95% confidence intervals of the sample means. However, intra-individual reproducibility of this approach has not been assessed, and is an important prerequisite for further implementing this approach.

In this chapter we describe polynomial analysis of ABPM data, and test the hypothesis that it is better reproducible the analysis of actual data and that this is so, not only with means of populations, but also with individual data. For the estimate of reproducibility duplicate standard errors as well as intra-class correlations were calculated of ABPM data from untreated mildly hypertensive patients who underwent ABPM for 24 hours twice, 1 week interval.

3. METHODS, STATISTICAL MODEL

Ten patients, 6 females/ 4 males, who had given their informed consent, participated in the study. Each patient had been examined at our outpatient clinic. Age varied from 33 to 52 years of age (mean 42 years), body mass index from 20 tp 31 kg/m (mean 29 kg/m). Patients were either housewife or actively employed throughout the study and had no other diseases. Previously treated patients had a washout period of at least 8 weeks before they were included in the study. All patients were included if untreated distolic blood pressure was repeatedly between 90 and 100 mm Hg and systolic blood pressure less than 170 mm Hg.

In all of the patients ABPM consisted of measurements every 60 minutes for 24 hours with a validated[7] light weight automated portable equipment (Space Lab Medical Inc, Redmond WA, model 90207). In the meantime patients performed their usual daily activities.

We define the dependent variable, the blood pressure recording at hour t, and, subsequently, model it as a function of hour t, hour t squared, hour t to the power 3, hour t to the power 4, and so on. The a's and b's are constants for the best fit of the given data, and are also called the regression weights.

Blood pressure at hour $t = a + b_1$ (hour t) $+ b_2$ (hour t) $^2 + b_3$ (hour t) $^3 + b_4$ (hour t) $^4 + ...$

If we use Fourier analysis instead the equation is

Blood pressure at hour t =

$p + q_1$ cos (hour t) $+..+ q_n$ cos n(hour t) $+ r_1$ sin (hour t) $+..+ r_n$ sin n(hour t)

with p, q_{1-n} and r_{1-n} being constants for the best fit of the given data.

Figure 1 shows the ambulatory blood pressure measurement (ABPM) systolic blood pressures in a patient with mild hypertension. During the daytime, blood pressure is much higher than at night, and this is the same on the second day. Bloosd pressure increases slowly to a maximum value at apporximately noon and then decreases to aminimum at approximately 6 p.m. The lower graph of the Figure shows the 4th order Fourier and polynomial graphs of these data (virtually the same). The goodness of fit as estimated by correlations between observed and modeled data (data not presented, but available from the authors) of a 4th order polynomial model appeared to be very good, and at least as good as the real sine-like function derived from the Fourier analysis. We, therefore, decided to choose out of the different lines the one with the smallest standard deviation (SD) of the points about the line. In our case the regression lines of the 4th and 7th orders generally provided the best fit for most of the samples. This is no surprise since particularly these equations provide the typical sinusoidal patterns, which circadian blood pressures are assumed to follow.[8] Actually, the 7th order polynome generally provided a slightly better fit than did the 4th order polynome and, so, we decided to routinely use this one.

STATISTICAL ANALYSIS

Reproducibility of ABPM was studied in the ten patients by performing 24 hour ABPM in each of them twice, intervals at least 1 week. Reproducibility of the duplicate data, as obtained, were assessed both by quantifying reproducibility on means of the population, and on the individual data.

REPRODUCIBILITY OF MEANS OF THE POPULATION

For this purpose we used duplicate standards error (Duplicate SE) and intra-class correlation (ρ).[8]

Duplicate SE was calculated according to Duplicate $SE = \sqrt{\sum (x_1 - x_2)^2 / 2n}$, where x_1 and x_2 are individual data during 1st and 2nd tests, and n= 240 (10 times 24 duplicate observations).

Intra-class correlation (ρ) are another approach for the estimate of replicability of repeated measures in one subject, and are calculated according to

$$\rho_1 = \frac{\sigma^2 \bar{x}_1 - \sigma^2 \bar{x}_2 / \bar{x}_1}{\sigma^2 \bar{x}_1}$$

where $\bar{x}_1$ and $\bar{x}_2$ are the means of the 240 values during test 1 and test 2 respectively, and $\sigma^2 \bar{x}_2 / \bar{x}_1$ is the variance of $\bar{x}_2$ given $\bar{x}_1$, and $\sigma^2 \bar{x}_1 = \sigma^2 \bar{x}_1 - (\bar{x}_1 - \bar{x}_2)^2 / 4$.

REPRODUCIBILITY OF INDIVIDUAL DATA

For this purpose we similarly used duplicate standards error (SE) and intra-class correlation (ρ).

Duplicate SE was calculated according to $SE = \sqrt{\sum (x_1 - x_2)^2 / 2n}$ where x_1 and x_2 are individual data during 1st and 2nd tests, and n= 24 (24 duplicate observations per patient).

Intra-class correlation (ρ) was calculated according to

$$\rho_1 = \frac{\sigma^2 \bar{x}_1 - \sigma^2 \bar{x}_2 / \bar{x}_1}{\sigma^2 \bar{x}_1}$$

where $\bar{x}_1$ and $\bar{x}_2$ are the means of the 24 values during test 1 and test 2 respectively, and $\sigma^2 \bar{x}_2 / \bar{x}_1$ is the variance of $\bar{x}_2$ given $\bar{x}_1$, and $\sigma^2 \bar{x}_1 = \sigma^2 \bar{x}_1 - (\bar{x}_1 - \bar{x}_2)^2 / 4$.

Calculations were performed using SPSS statistical software, polynomial curves were drawn using Harvard Graphics 3.[9,10] Under the assumption of standard deviations of 25 % and intraclass correlations of + 0.7, at least 240 duplicate observations had to be included to obtain a regression analysis with a statistical power of 80% and a 5 % significance level. And so, it seemed appropriate to include hourly data of at least 10 patients tested twice for 24 hours. Paired data, Duplicate SE and intraclass correlation were statistically tested by t-tests, F-tests, or McNemar's chi-square tests, whenever appropriate.

4. RESULTS

REPRODUCIBILITY OF MEANS OF POPULATION

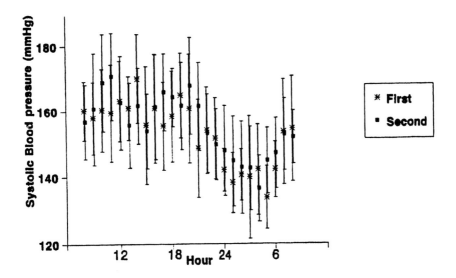

Fig. 1   Mean values of ABPM data of 10 untreated patients with mild hypertension ands their SDs,   recorded twice, one week in-between.

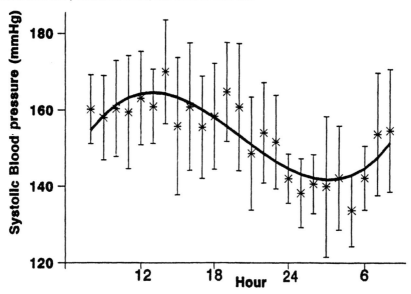

Fig. 2   Polynome of corresponding ABPM recording (first one) from Fig. 1, reflecting a clear circadian rhythm of systolic blood pressures.

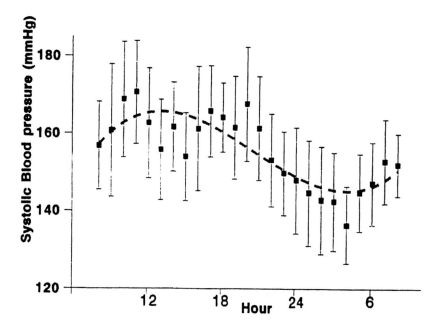

Fig. 3 *Polynome of corresponding ABPM recording (second one) from Fig. 1, again reflecting a clear circadian rhythm of systolic blood pressures.*

Figure 1 shows mean values of ABPM of 10 untreated patients and their SDs, recorded twice, one week in-between. Obviously, there is an enormous variance in the data both between-subject and within-subject as demonstrated respectively by the large SDs and the considerable differences between means. Figure 2 and 3 give polynomes of corresponding data from figure 1, reflecting a clear circadian rhythm in systolic blood pressures. Fig. 4 shows that the two polynomes are, obviously, very much similar. Within-subject tests for reproducibility are given in Table I. Duplicate SEs of means versus zero and versus grand mean were 15.9 and 7.2, while of polynomes they were only 1.86 (differences in Duplicate SEs significant at a $P<0.001$ level). Intra-class correlations (ρs) of means versus zero and versus grand mean were 0.46 and 0.75, while of polynomes they were 0.986 (differences in levels of correlation significant at a $P<0.001$). Obviously, polynomes of ABPM data of means of populations produce significantly better reproducibility, than do the actual data.

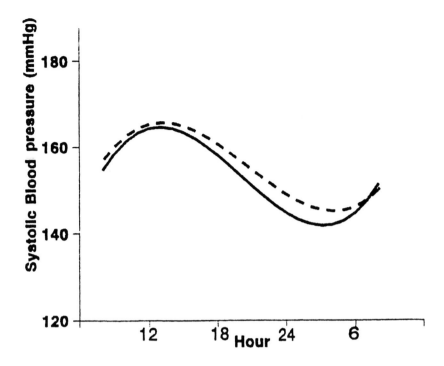

Fig. 4   The two polynomes from Figs. 2 and 3 are, obviously, very much similar.

CHAPTER 10

Table 1

24 hr ambulatory blood pressure measurements in a group of 10 patients with untreated mild hypertension tested twice: reproducibility of means of population.

	mean values variations vs zero	mean values variations vs grand mean	polynomes
Means (mm Hg) (test 1 / test 2)	153.1 / 155.4	153.1 / 155.4	-
SD (σ) (mm Hg) (test 1 / test 2)	21.9 / 21.1	15.7 / 13.8	-
95 % CIs[1] (mm Hg) (test 1 / test 2)	139.4-166.8/142.2-168.6	143.3-163.9/146.8-164.0	-
Differences between means (SD, σ) (mm Hg)	-2.4 (22.4)	-2.3 (10.5)	-
P values differences between results tests 1 and 2	0.61	0.51	0.44
Duplicate SEs[2] (mm Hg)	15.9	7.2	1.86
Relative Duplicate SEs[3] (%)	66	31	7
Intra-class correlations[4] (ρs)	0.46	0.75	0.986
95 % CIs	0.35-0.55	0.26-0.93	0.972-0.999
Proportion total variance responsible for between-patient variance (%)	46	75	99
95 % CIs (%)	35-55	26-93	97-100

[1] CIs = confidence intervals.
[2] Duplicate SEs calculated according to Duplicate SE = $\sqrt{ \Sigma (x_1-x_2)^2 / 2n }$, where x_1 and x_2 are individual data during 1st and 2nd test, and n=240 (10 times 24 duplicate observations) .
[3] Calculated as 100%x[Duplicate SD/ (overall mean – 130 mm Hg)].
[4] Intra-class correlations ($ρ_1$ s) calculated according to

$$\rho_1 = \frac{\sigma^2 \overline{X}_1 - \sigma^2 \overline{X}_2 / \overline{X}_1}{\sigma^2 \overline{X}_1}$$

where $\overline{X}_1$ and $\overline{X}_2$ are the means of the 240 values during test 1 and test 2 respectively, and $\sigma^2 \overline{X}_2 / \overline{X}_1$ is the variance of $\overline{X}_2$ given $\overline{X}_1$, and $\sigma^2 \overline{X}_2 / \overline{X}_1 = \sigma^2 \overline{X}_1 - (\overline{X}_1 - \overline{X}_2)^2 / 4.$

REPRODUCIBILITY OF INDIVIDUAL DATA

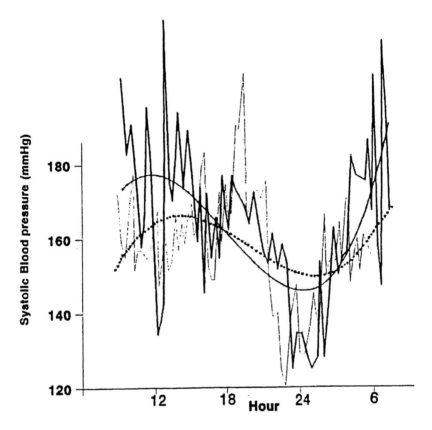

Fig. 5   *Individual data from patient 1 (Table 2) during first ABPM (fat line) and second ABPM recording (thin line). The corresponding polynomes of the two recordings (continuous and dotted curves respectively) are somewhat more different from each other than are the differences between the group data polynomes (Fig. 4). Yet, they offer much better similarity than do the actual data.*

Table 2

24 hr ambulatory blood pressure measurements in 10 patients with untreated mild hypertension tested twice: reproducibility of individual data.

Patient	mean (mm Hg) test 1 / test 2	SD (mm Hg) test 1 / test 2	Duplicate SEs (mm Hg) [1]		Intraclass Correlations[2]	
			raw data	polynomes	raw data	polynomes
1	160 / 157	14 / 18	17.7	2.1	0.07	0.58
2	158 / 161	17 / 27	17.6	9.0	0.27	0.53
3	160 / 169	20 / 29	19.7	2.6	-0.23	0.03
4	159 / 171	23 / 21	19.1	7.2	0.11	0.29
5	163 / 163	19 / 23	19.7	9.9	0.10	0.20
6	161 / 156	15 / 20	21.4	6.4	0.03	0.10
7	170 / 162	21 / 18	10.1	8.2	0.57	0.70
8	156 / 154	28 / 18	6.3	6.7	0.26	0.24
9	161 / 161	26 / 25	18.2	13.5	0.60	0.81
10	155 / 166	21 / 19	11.9	6.6	0.53	0.96

pooled data

	153.1 / 155.4	21.9 / 21.1	$16.2(5.0)^3$	7.2(3.3)	0.26(0.26)	0.42(0.34)
			___ P<0.001 ___		___ P=0.009 ___	

[1] Duplicate SEs calculated according to $SE = \sqrt{\sum\limits^{n} (x_1-x_2)^2 / 2n}$, where x_1 and x_2 are individual data during 1st and 2nd test, and n= 24 (24 duplicate observations per patient).

[2] Intra-class correlations (ρs) calculated according to

$$\rho_i = \frac{\sigma^2 \overline{X}_1 - \sigma^2 \overline{X}_2 / \overline{X}_1}{\sigma^2 \overline{X}_1}$$

where $\overline{X}_1$ and $\overline{X}_2$ are the means of the 24 values during test 1 and test 2 respectively, and $\sigma^2 \overline{X}_2 / \overline{X}_1$ is the variance of $\overline{X}_2$ given $\overline{X}_1$, and $\sigma^2 \overline{X}_2 / \overline{X}_1 = \sigma^2 \overline{X}_1 - (\overline{X}_1 - \overline{X}_2)^2 / 4$.

[3] SDs between the brackets.

Figure 5 gives an example of the individual data of patient no. 1 during the first and second test and also shows his corresponding polynomes of test 1 and test 2. Although, again, there is enormous variability in the data, the polynomes have rather similar patterns. Table II gives an overview of assessments of reproducibility for each patient separately. Duplicate SEs of raw data were generally more than twice the size of those of the polynomes, while intraclass correlations of the actual data were accordingly generally almost half the size of those of the polynomes with median values of 0.26 and 0.38 and ranges between –0.23 and 0.60 and between 0.03 and 0.96 respectively. Pooled differences were highly significant both for the

Duplicate SEs, and for the intraclass correlations (P<0.001 and P=0.009 respectively, Table II).

5. DISCUSSION

In this paper we demonstrate that ABPM systolic blood pressures in untreated mildly hypertensive patients can be readily assessed by polynomial analysis and that this approach unlike the actual data analysis is highly reproducible. Similar results were obtained when instead of systolic blood pressures diastolic or mean pressures were analyzed. It may be argued from a mathematical-statistical point of view that the better reproducibility is a direct consequence of the procedure where variability is reduced by taking means of a population rather than individual values. However, when we compared polynomial and actual data for each subject separately, although the overall level of reproducibility fell, the former approach still performed better than did the latter. This indicates that the better reproducibility may at least in part be connected with mechanisms other than the mathematical necessity of reducing variability by taking the polynomial modeling of the actual data. Particularly, polynomes may be better reproducible, because they are a better estimate of the circadian rhythm of blood pressure than the actual data, which are of course influenced by a variety of exogenic factors including daily activities, meals and breaks, psychological effects. A polynome would be a more accurate estimate of the true endogenic circadian rhythm, where the mathematical procedure takes care that exogenic factors are largely removed. This would explain the high reproducibility not only of polynomial analyses of population data but also of individual patient data.

Polynomial analysis has been validated in chronobiology, as a reproducible method for the study of circadian rhythms in normotensive subjects, and is, actually, routinely used for that purpose in the Department of Chronobiology of our academic hospital.[11,12] So far, however, it has received little attention in the clinical assessment of patients with hypertension. The current paper suggests, that the method would be a reliable instrument for that purpose.

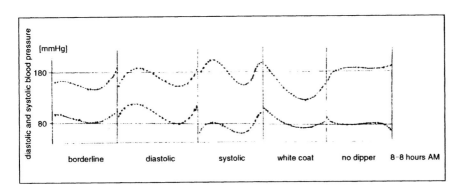

Fig. 6 Polynomial analysis can be used to identify circadian patterns of blood pressure in individual patients.

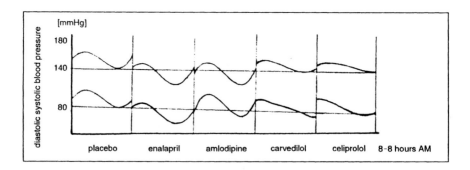

Fig. 7 Polynomial analysis can be used to study the effects of antihypertensive drugs in groups of patients.

Polynomial analysis, could, e.g., be used to identify circadian patterns of blood pressure in individual patients. Figure 6 gives an example of 5 such patterns readily demonstrable by polynomes. These polynomes were drawn from ABPM data from our own outpatient clinic database. Figure 7 gives another example of how polynomes can be helpful in clinical assessments. The polynomes present the mean results of a recent study by our group, comparing the short term effects of different blood pressure reducing agents in mildly hypertensive patients (n=10).[6] All of the polynomes were within 95% CIs of the mean data of our samples. Differences between the data in this study, as assessed by 2-way analysis of variance, established that on enalapril, and amlodipine, unlike beta-blockers carvedilol and celiprolol, time effect was a major source of variability. The polynomes visualized that this was so, because beta-blockers did not reduce nighttime blood pressures. So, polynomial analysis was helpful in interpreting the results of this study. We conclude that polynomial analysis of ABPM data, unlike actual data analysis, is highly reproducible in patients with mild hypertension, and that this is so not only with population means but also with individual data. It is, therefore, a valid approach for the clinical assessment of hypertensive patients, and may, thus, be helpful for a variety of purposes, e.g., for identifying circadian patterns of blood pressure in individual patients, and for the study of antihypertensive drugs in groups of patients.

6. REFERENCES

1.   Owens P, Lyons S, O'Brien E. Ambulatory blood pressure in hypertensive population: patterns and prevalence of hypertensive subforms. J Hypertens 1998; 16: 1735-1745.
2.   Zanchetti A. Twenty-four-hour ambulatory blood pressure evaluation of antihypertensive agents. J Hypertens 1997; 15: S21-S25.

3. Omboni S, Parati G, Palatini P, Vanasia A, Muiesan ML, Cuspidi C, Mancia
    G. Reproducibility and clinical value of nocturnal hypotension: prospective
    evidence from the SAMPLE study. J Hypertens 1998; 16: 733 -738.
4. Bleniaszewski L, Staessen JA, Byttebier G, De Leeuw PW, Van Hedent T,
    Fagard R. Trough-to-peak versus surface ration in the assessment of
    antihypertensive agents. Blood Press 1997; 4: 350-357.
5. Van de Luit L, Van der Meulen J, Cleophas TJ, Zwinderman AH. Amplified
    amplitudes of circadian rhythms and nighttime hypotension in patients with
    chronic fatigue syndrome; improvement by inopamil but not by melatonin.
    Eur J Intern Med 1998; 9: 99-103.
6. Van de Luit L, Cleophas TJ, Van der Meulen J, Zwinderman AH. Nighttime
    hypotension in mildly hypertensive patients prevented by beta-blockers but
    not by ACE-inhibitors or calcium channel blockers. Eur J Intern Med 1998; 9:
    251-256.
7. O'Brien E, Atkins N, Staessen J. State of the market, a review of ambulatory
    blood pressure-monitoring devices. Hypertension 1995; 26: 835-842.
8. Hays WL. Curvilinear regression. In: Hays WL, Statistics, Holt, Rinehart and
    Winston, Inc, Chicago, 4th edition, 1988, pp 698-716.
9. SPSS. Statistical Software. Professional Statistics. Chicago, Ill, 1996.
10. Harvard Graphics-3. Statistical Software. Boston MA, Harvard, Inc, 1995.
11. Scheidel B, Lemmer B, Blume H. Influence of time of day on
    pharmacokinetics and hemodynamic effects of beta-blockers. In: Clinical
    Chronopharmacology. Munich, Germany: Zuckschwerdt Verlag, 1990; vol 6:
    75-9.
12. Lemmer B, Scheidel B, Behne S. Chronopharmacokinetics and
    chronopharmacodynamics of cardiovascular active drugs: propranolol, organic
    nitrates, nifedipine. Ann NY Acad Sci 1991; 618: 166-171.

CHAPTER 11

META-ANALYSIS

1. INTRODUCTION

Problems with meta-analyses are frequent: regressions are often nonlinear; effects are often multivariate rather than univariate; continuous data frequently have to be transformed into binary data for the purpose of comparibility; bad studies may be included; coverage may be limited; data may not be homogeneous; failure to relate data to hypotheses may obscure discrepancies. In spite of these well-recognized flaws, the method of meta-analysis is an invaluable scientific activity: Meta-analyses establish whether scientific findings are consistent and can be generalized across populations and treatment variations, or whether findings vary significantly between particular subsets. Explicit methods used limit bias and improve reliability and accuracy of conclusions, and increase the power and precision of estimates of treatment effects and risk exposures. In the past decade, despite reservations on the part of regulatory bodies, the method of meta-analysis has increasingly been employed in drug development programs for the purpose of exploration of changes in treatment effect over time, integrated summaries of safety and efficacy of new treatments, integrating existing information, providing data for rational decision making, and even prospective planning in drug development.

Meta-analyses are increasingly considered an integral part of phase III drug research programs for two reasons. First, meta-analysis of existing data instead of an unsystematic literature search before starting a phase III drug trial has been documentedly helpful in defining the hypothesis to be tested. Second, although meta-analyses are traditionally considered post-hoc analyses that do not test the primary hypotheses of the data, they do test hypotheses that are extremely close to the primary ones. It may be argued, therefore, that with the established uniform guidelines as proposed by Oxman and Guyatt and implemented by the Cochrane Collaborators, probability statements are almost as valid as they are in completely randomized controlled trials.

Meta-analyses should be conducted under the collective responsibility of experienced clinicians and biostatisticians familiar with relevant mathematical approaches. They may still be improved, by a combination of experience and theory, to the point at which findings can be taken as sufficiently reliable where there is no other analysis or confirmation is available.

Meta-analyses depend upon quantity and quality of original research studies as reported. Helpful initiatives to both ends include the Unpublished Paper Amnesty Movement endorsed by the editors of nearly 100 international journals in September 1997 which will help to reduce the quantity of unpublished papers, and the Consolidated Standards of Reporting Trials (CONSORT) Statement (1997) developed by high impact journals which is concerned with quality and standardization of submitted papers.

Meta-analysis can help reduce uncertainty, prevent unnecessary repetition of costly research, and shorten the time between research discoveries and clinical implementation of effective diagnostic and therapeutic treatments, but it can only do so when its results are made available. The continuously updated Cochrane Database of Systematic Reviews on the Internet is an excellent example for that purpose. Medical journals including specialist journals have a responsibility of their own. So much so that they may be able to lead the way for biased experts, who are so convinced of their own biased experience and so little familiar with meta-analysis.

2. EXAMPLES

We have come a long way since psychologists in the early 70s drew attention to the systematic steps needed to minimize biases and random errors in reviews of research. E.g., we currently have wonderful meta-analyses of pharmacological treatments for cardiovascular diseases which helped us very much to make proper listings of effective treatments (as well as less effective ones). So, now we are able to answer 1st what is best for our patients, 2nd how we should distribute our resources. For example, for acute myocardial infarction, thrombolytic therapy as well as aspirin are highly effective, while lidocaine and calcium channel blockers are not so. For secondary prevention myocardial infarction cholesterol-reducing therapy were highly effective while other therapies were less so or were even counterproductive, e.g., class I antiarrhythmic agents as demonstrated in Figure 1).

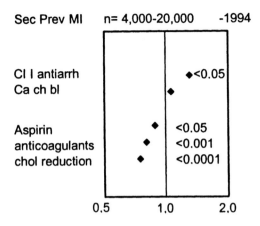

Fig. 1. Pooled results (Odds ratios = odds of infarction in treated subjects / odds of infarction in controls) of secundary prevention trials heart infarction.

Currently, even epidemiologists are borrowing from clinical pharmacologists and clinical investigators, and they are quite successful in showing the likeliness of various epidemiological issues such as the epidemiology of various cardiovascular conditions. It should be emphasized that the logic behind meta-analysis is simple and straightforward. All it requires, is to stick to the scientific methods, that is (1) a clearly defined prior hypothesis, (2) thorough search of trials, (3) strict inclusion criteria for trials, and (4) uniform guidelines for data analysis.

3. CLEARLY DEFINED HYPOTHESES

In chapter 1 we discussed that drug trials principally addres efficacy and safety of new drugs. It is specified in advance –in the statistical analysis plan- what are the main outcome variables, and how they should be tested.

A meta-analysis is very much similar to a single trial, and similarly to a single trial it tests a very small number of primary hypotheses, mostly the hypotheses that the new compound is more efficaceous and safe than the reference compound. This implies that data dredging is as unacceptable for meta-analyses as it is for separate clinical trials.

4. THOROUGH SEARCH OF TRIALS

The activity of thoroughly searching-published-research requires a systematic procedure. E.g., searching medline requires a whole lot of tricks, and has to be learned. Unless you already know, you may pick up a checklist for this purpose, similarly to the checklist used by aircraft staff before take off, a nice simile used by Dr Oxman from McMasters University, one of the enlightened specialists of meta-analyses. A faulty review of trials is as perilous as a faulty aircraft and both of them are equally deadly, the former particularly so if we are going to use it for making decisions about health care. Search terms will soon put you on the right track when searching medline.   SH, e.g., means "subject-heading" which is controlled vocabulary; TW means "free-text-word" (searching with a lot of TWs increases sensitivity but reduces specificity of the search. There are sensitive ways to look for RCTs. ADJ is another TW and is more precise than AND. NOT means that first and third step are combined and second step is excluded. Using checklists consistent of search terms of controlled vocabulary and frequently use free text words makes things   so   much   easier   and   overcomes   the   risk   of   being   unsuccesful.

5. STRICT INCLUSION CRITERIA

The third scientific rule is strict inclusion criteria. Inclusion criteria are concerned with validity of the trials to be included, which means their likeliness of being unbiased. Strict inclusion criteria means that we subsequently only include the valid studies. A valid study is an unbiased study , a study that is unlikely to include systematic errors. The most dangerous error in reviews are systematic errors otherwise called biases. Checking validity is thus the most important thing both for doers and for users of systematic reviews. Some factors have empirically been shown to beneficially influence validity. These factors include: blinding the study; random assignment of patients; explicit description of methods; accurate statistics; accurate ethics including written informed consent.

6. UNIFORM DATA ANALYSIS

Statistical analysis is a tool which, when used appropriately, can help us to derive meaningful conclusions from the data. And it can help us to avoid analytic errors. Statistics should be simple and should test primary hypotheses in the first place. Before any analysis or plotting of data can be performed we have to decide what kind of data we have.

1.INDIVIDUAL DATA

Meta-analyses of primary data of previously published studies are generally not accessible for use. Usually we have to accept the summary statistics from studies instead. This is of course less informative and less precise than a synthesis of primary data but can still provide useful information.

2. CONTINUOUS DATA MEANS AND SEMS

We just take the mean result of the mean difference of the outcome variable we want to meta-analyze and add up. The data can be statistically tested according to unpaired t-test of the sum of multiple means

$$t = \frac{mean_1 + mean_2 + mean_3 \ldots}{\sqrt{SEM_1{}^2 + SEM_2{}^2 + SEM_3{}^2 + \ldots}}$$

with degrees of freedom $= n_1 + n_2 + n_3 + \ldots n_k - k$

3. PROPERTIONS: RELATIVE RISKS (RRS), ODDS RATIOS (ORS), DIFFERENCES BETWEEN RELATIVE RISKS (RDS)

Probably, 99% of meta-analyses make use of proportions rather than continuous data, even if original studies provided predominantly the latter particularly for efficacy data (mean fall in blood pressure etc.). This is so both for efficacy and safety meta-analyses. Sometimes data have to be remodeled from quantitative into binary ones for that purpose.

Calculation of point estimates and their variances

Contingency table	numbers of patients with disease improvement	numbers of patients with no improvement	total
test treatment	a	b	a+b
reference treatment	c	d	c+d
total	a+c	b+d	n

Point estimators RR, OR, or RD:
RR= a/(a+b) / c/(c+d)
OR= a/b / c/d
RD= a/(a+b) - c/(c+d)

The data can be statistically tested by use of a chi-square test of the added point estimators.
Instead of RR and OR we take lnRR and lnOR in order to approximate normality

$$Chi\text{-}square = \frac{LnRR_1/s_1{}^2 + lnRR_2/s_2{}^2 + lnRR_3/s_3{}^2 \ldots}{1/s_1{}^2 + 1/s_2{}^2 + 1/s_3{}^2 + \ldots}$$

degrees of freedom 1 (one).

s^2 = variance of point estimate :
$s_{lnRR}{}^2 = 1/a - 1/(a+b) + 1/c - 1/(c+d)$
$s_{lnOR}{}^2 = 1/a + 1/b + 1/c + 1/d$
$s_{RV}{}^2 = ab/(a+b)^3 + cd/(c+d)^3$

for RV, which does not have so much skewed a distribution, ln-transformation is
not needed.

$$\text{Chi-square} = \frac{RV_1/s_1^2 + RV_2/s_2^2 + RV_3/s_3^2 + ...}{1/s_1^2 + 1/s_2^2 + 1/s_3^2 + ...}$$

As alternative approach Mantel-Haenszl-summary chi-square can be used:

Mantel-Haenszl summary chi-square test:

$$a_1d_1/n_1 + a_2d_2/n_2 + a_3d_3/n_3 + ... / \quad b_1c_1/n_1 + b_2c_2/n_2 + b_3c_3/n_3 ...... = (\Sigma ad/n) / \Sigma(bc/n)$$

This approach has been explained in chapter 3. Results of the two approaches yield
similar results. However, with Mantel-Haenszl the calculation of pooled variances
is rather complex, and a computer program is required.
A good starting point with any statistical analysis is plotting the data.

PUBLICATION BIAS

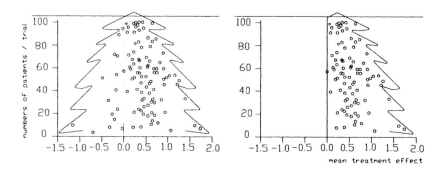

*Fig. 2. This christmas tree otherwise called funnel plot of 100 published trials
shows on the x-axis the mean result of each trial; on the y-axis it shows the
numbers of pts involved in each trial. As you can see on the left, there is a
christmas-tree or upside- down-funnel-pattern of distribution of the results. The
smaller the trial, the larger the distribution of results. Right graph gives a
simulated pattern, suggestive for **publication bias**: the negative trials are not
published and thus missing. This cut christmas-tree can help us suspect that there
is a considerable publication bias in the meta- analysis.*

This socalled funnel plot of 100 published trials shows on the x-axis the mean result of each trial; on the y-axis it shows the numbers of pts involved in each trial. As you can see on the left, there is a christmas-tree or upside-down-funnel-pattern of distribution of the results. The smaller the trial, the larger the distribution of results. Right graph gives a simulated pattern, suggestive for publication bias: the negative trials are not published and thus missing. This cut christmas-tree can help us suspect that there is a considerable publication bias in the meta-analysis. Publication bias can also be statistically tested by by rank correlation between variances and odds ratios. If small studies with negative results are less likely to be published, rank correlation would be high, if not it would be low (Kendall tau test).

KENDALL TAU TEST

Normally correlation coefficient r measures actual results. Tau-test basically does the same, but uses ranked data instead of actual data.

Trial   A B C D E F G H I
Ranknumber of size 1 2 3 4 5 6 7 8 9 10
of trial
Ranknumber of size 5 3 1 4 2 7 9 6 10 8
of mean result

Lower row add up ranknumbers higher than 5, resp 3, resp 1, resp 4: we find
$5+6+7+5+5+3+1+2+0+0=34$
Then lower row add up ranknumbers lower than 5, 3, 1, etc: we find
$4+2+0+1+0+1+2+0+1+0=11$
As standard error of this result is $\sqrt{n(n-1)(2n+5)/18}$ and as we may assume a normal distribution. We can now test this correlation and find $(34-11)/\sqrt{n(n-1)(2n+5)/18}= 1.968$ which is approximately $1.96=2=$is the number of SEMs distant from which is $\leq 5\%$ of the data. And so, the null hypothesis of no publication bias has to be rejected. Publication bias can also be tested by calculating the shift of odds ratios caused by adding of unpublished trials e.g. from abstract-reports or proceedings.

HETEROGENEITY

Figure 3 gives an example of a meta-analysis with means and 95% CIs, telling us something about heterogeneity.

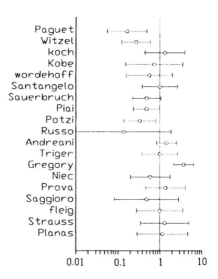

Fig. 3. Heterogeneous trials. On the x-axis is the result, on the y-axis are the trials.
We see the results of 19 trials of endoscopic sclerotherapy for esophageal bleeding

On the x-axis is the result, on the y-axis are the trials. This example has been previously used by Dr Thompson from London School of Hygiene and Tropical Medicine. We see the results of 19 trials of endoscopic sclerotherapy for esophageal varices bleeding: odds ratios less than one represent a beneficial effect. These trials were considerably different in pt-selection, baseline-severity-of-condition, slerotechniques, management-of –bleeding-otherwise, and duration-of-follow-up. And so, this is a meta-analysis which is clinically very heterogeneous. Is it also statistically heterogeneous? For that purpose we test whether there is a greater variation between the results of the trials than is compatible with the play of chance, simply using a chi-square test. In so doing, we find $\chi^2 = 43$ for 19-1=18 dfs. The p value is <.001 giving substantial evidence for statistical heterogeneity. For the interpretation of such tests it is useful to know that a χ^2 statistic has on average a value equal to the degrees of freedom, so a result of $\chi^2 = 18$ with 18 dfs would give no evidence for heterogeneity, values much larger such as here observed do so for the opposite.

With very few studies in the meta-analysis, or with small studies, the socalled fixed model approach has little power, and is susceptible to type II errors of not finding heterogeneity which may actually be in the data.

A little bit better power is then provided by the random effect model of Dersimonian and Laird, which assumes an additional variable. The variable $s_{between\ trials}$ is added to the model, meaning the size of variance between the trials. Table 1 shows the mathematical model.

Table 1

Mathematical models for testing the presence of heterogeneity of ordinal data (for continuous data multiple group ANOVA may be used).

Fixed effect model

test for homogeneity
$$\chi^2 = [RV_1^2/s_1^2 + RV_2^2/s_2^2 + RV_3/s_3^2 \ldots$$
$$-(RV_1/s_1^2 + RV_2/s_2^2 + RV_3/s_3^2 ..)] / (1/s_1^2 + 1/s_2^2 + 1/s_3^2 + ..)$$

Random effect model (DerSimonian and Laird)

Test for heterogeneity is identical, except for variances s^2 which are replaced by $(s^2 + s_{between\ trials}^2)$.

Example of Random effect model analysis

trial	test treatment		reference treatment	
	deaths	survivors	deaths	survivors
1	1	24	5	20
2	5	95	15	85
3	25	475	50	450

In the above example, the test for heterogeneity fixed effect model provides $\chi^2 = 1.15$ with dfs 3-1=2, while the test with the random effect model provides a $\chi^2 = 1.29$ with dfs equally 2, both lower than 2. The between-trial variance $s_{between\ trials}^2$ is thus accepted to be zero and the weights of the two models are equal. Heterogeneity can be neglected. With the simple example given, the two approaches to test homogeneity raise similar results(the null hypothesis is tested that studies are equal). And so, between-trial variance $s_{between\ trials}^2$ is accepted to be zero and theresults of the two models are equal.
Heterogeneity can be neglected in this example.

HETEROGENEITY AND SUB-GROUP ANALYSIS

When there is heterogeneity, to doers of systematic reviews, that's when things first get really exciting. A careful investigation of the potential cause of heterogeneity has to be accomplished. The main focus then should be on trying to understand any sources of heterogeneity in the data. In practice, this may be less hard to assess since the doers have frequently noticed clinical differences already, and it thus becomes relatively easy to test the data accordingly. Figure 4 below shows how age e.g. is a determinant of illness, but in the right graph the risk difference is heterogeneous because it increases with age.

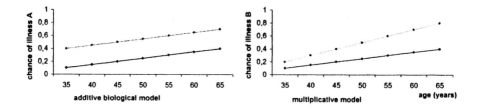

Fig. 4. Age is a determinant of illness, but in the right graph the risk difference is heterogeneous because it increases with age.

Except age, outliers may give an important clue about the cause of heterogeneity.

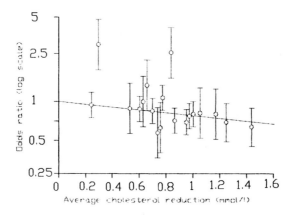

Fig. 5. The relation between cholesterol and coronary heart disease. The two outliers on top were the main cause for heterogeneity in the data: one study was different because it achieved a very small reduction of cholesterol; the other was a very short- term study.

Figure 5 shows the relation between cholesterol and coronary heart disease. The two outliers on top were the main cause for heterogeneity in the data: one study was different because it achieved a very small reduction of cholesterol; the other was a very shortterm study.

Still other causes of heterogeneity may be involved. 33 Studies of cholesterol and risk of carcinomas showed that heterogeneity was huge. When the trials were divided according to social class, the effect in the lowest class was 4 -5 times those of the middle and upper class,

explaining everything about this heterogeneous result.

We should of course warn of the danger of overinterpretation of heterogeneity. Heterogeneity may occur by chance. This is particularly an important possibility to consider when no clinical explanation is found. Also, we should warn that a great deal of uniformity among the results of independently performed studies is not necessarily good; it can suggest consistency-in-bias rather than consistency-in-real-effects.

TESTING ROBUSTNESS OF THE DATA AT THE COMPLETION OF DATA ANALYSIS

Sensitivity or robustness of a meta-analysis is one last important aspect to be addressed in the analysis of the data. When talking of strict inclusion criteria, we discussed studies with lower levels of validity, as assessed by factors such as blinding, random assignments, accurate and explicit description of results and statistics. It may be worthwhile not to completely reject the studies with lower methodology. They can be used for assessing another characteristic of meta-analyses, namely its sensitivity.

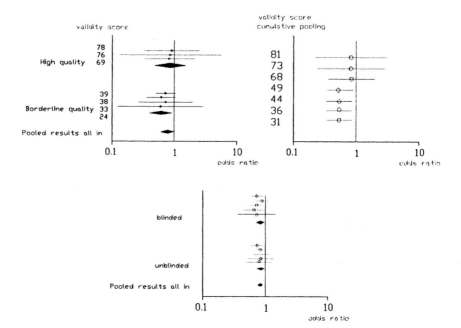

Fig. 6. The left upper graph gives an example of how the pooled data of three high-quality-studies provide a smaller result, than do 4 studies-of-borderline-quality. The summary result is mainly determined by the borderline-quality-studies, as is also shown in the cumulative-right-upper -graph. When studies are ordered according to their being blinded or not as shown in the lower graph, differences may be large or may be not so. In studies using objective variables, eg blood pressures, heart rates, blinding is not so important than in studies using subjective variables (pain scores etc). In this particular example differences were negligible.

This left upper graph (Figure 6) gives an example of how the pooled data of three high-quality-studies provide a smaller result, than do 4 studies-of-borderline-quality. The summary result is mainly determined by the borderline-quality-studies, as is also shown in the cumulative-right-upper -graph. When studies are ordered according to their being blinded or not as shown in the lower graph, differences may be large or may be not so. In studies using objective variables, eg blood pressures, heart rates, blinding is not so important than in studies using subjective variables (pain scores etc). In this particular example differences were negligible.So, in conclusion, when examining the influence of various inclusion criteria on the overall odds ratios, we may come to conclude that the criteria themselves are an important factor in determining the summary result. We say in that case that the meta-analysis lacks robustness (otherwise called sensitivity or precision of point estimates). Interpretation then has to be cautious, pooling may have to be left out altogether. Just leaving out trials at this stage of the meta-analysis is inappropriate either, because it would introduce bias similar to publication-bias or bias-introduced-by-not-complying-with-the-intention-to-treat-principle.

7. DISCUSSION, WHERE ARE WE NOW?

Several recent publications were critical of the method of meta-analysis: e.g., Chalmers and Lau in JAMA 1996 and Lelorier in NEJM 1997 concluded that meta-analyses did not accurately predict the outcomes of subsequent large trials. Colditz and Berlin JAMA 1999 concluded that meta-analyses were not or at least not-yet good enough to identify adverse drug reactions. Why so? Probably, the answer is (1st) trials must get better, and (2nd) publication bias must disappear altogether. There are several important initiatives being taken at this very moment that may be helpful to this aim. In May 1998 editors of 70 journals have endorsed the Consolidated- Standards-of-Reporting-Trials-Statement (the socalled CONSORT-Statement) developed by JAMA, BMJ, Lancet, and Annals-of-Int- Med in an effort to standardize the way trials are reported, with special-emphasis on the-intention-to-treat-principle in order to reduce treatment-related selection-bias. For investigators, <reporting> according to such standards will become much easier, and will even become a non-issue if requirements as requested by CONSORT are met. This initiative may have important potential to improve the level of validity of trials and thus facilitate their suitability for meta-analyses. Another important milestone is the initiative of the Unpublished-Paper-Amnesty-Movement. In September 1997 the editors of nearly 100 international journals invited investigators to submit unpublished study data in the form of unreported-trial-registration-forms. Submitted materials are routinely made availalble to the world through listing the trial-details on the journals'web sites, in addition to other ways. The International-Committee-of-Medical-Editors and the World-Association-of-Medical-Editors are currently helping these initiatives by standardizing the peer review system and training referees.

Where do we go? We go for the aim of meta-analyses being accepted as gold standard for :

1. Reporting randomized experimental research.
2. Setting the stage for the development of new drugs.
3. Determination of individual therapies.
4. Leading the way for regulatory organs.
5. Maybe soon even epidemiological research.

We will only accomplish these efforts if we stick to the scientific method, which we summed up for you earlier. However, today many meta-analyses are presented or published, that do not follow these simple scientific principles, and that just leave out validity assessment of trials included, or tests for heterogeneity and publication bias. Both journal editors and readers of meta-analyses must be critical and alert since a flawed meta-analysis of unreliable and biased material is deadly, not only to research but also to health care. The above guidelines enable not only to perform meta-analyses but also to identify flawed meta-analyses, and, more importantly, to identify and appreciate well-performed meta-analyses.

8. REFERENCES

1. Chalmers I, Altman DG.Systematic reviews. BMJ Publishing Group, London, UK, 1995.
2. Cleophas TJ. Human experimentation. Kluwer Academic Publishers, Dordrecht, Neth, 1999.

CHAPTER 12

CROSSOVER STUDIES WITH CONTINUOUS VARIABLES: POWER ANALYSIS

1. SUMMARY

Background: The crossover design is a sensitive means of determining the efficacy of new drugs because it eliminates between subject-variability. However, when the response in the first period carries on into the second (carryover effects) or when time factors can not be kept constant in a lengthy crossover (time effects), the statistical power of testing may be jeopardized. We recently demonstrated that the crossover design with binary variables is a powerful method in spite of such factors as carryover effects. Power analysis of crossover trials with continuous variables have not been explicitly studied.

Objective: Using the Grizzle model for the assessment of treatment effect, carryover effect and time effect, we drew power curves of hypothesized crossover studies with different levels of correlation between drug reponse.

Results: We demonstrate that the sensitivity of testing is largely dependent on the levels of correlation between drug response. Whenever the correlation coefficient is >0, we soon will have better sensitivity to test treatment effect than carryover effect or time effect of similar size. Whenever levels of correlation are not strong positive or negative the statistical power to demonstrate similarly-sized treatment and carryover effect, or treatment and time effect is approximately 80%, which is an acceptable level for reliable testing.

Conclusions: The crossover design is a powerful method for assessing positively correlated treatment comparisons, despite the risk of carryover and time effects.

2. INTRODUCTION

Crossover studies with continuous variables are routinely used in clinical drug research: for example, no less than 22% of the double-blind placebo-controlled hypertension trials in 1993 were accordingly designed.[1] A major advantage of the crossover design is that it eliminates between-subject variability of symptoms. However, problems include the occurrence of treatment-by-period interaction, otherwise called carryover effect (if the effect of the first period carries on into the next one, then it may influence the response to the latter period). Second, the possibility of time effects due to external factors such as the change of the seasons has to be taken into account in lengthy crossover studies. Third, negative correlations between drug response, although recently recognized in clinical pharmacology, is an important possibility not considered in the design and analysis of clinical trials so far. Many crossover studies may have a positive correlation-between-drug-response, not only because treatments in a given comparison are frequently from the same class of drugs, but also because one subject is used for comparisons of two treatments. Still, in treatment comparisons of completely different treatments patients may fall into different populations, those who respond better to the test-treatment and those who do so to the reference-treatment. This phenomenon has already lead to treatment protocols based on individualized rather than stepped care.[2] Power analyses for crossover studies with continuous variables so far only accounted for the possibility of approximately zero levels of correlations.[3-8] While considering different levels of correlation, we recently demonstrated[9] that the crossover design with binary variables is a powerful means of determining the efficacy of new drugs in spite of such factors as carryover effects. Crossover trials with continuous variables, however, have not yet been similarly studied.

In the current communication while taking both positive and negative correlations into account we drew power curves of hypothesized crossover studies with different amounts of treatment effect, carryover effect and time effect.

3. MATHEMATICAL MODEL

According to Scheffé[10] the notion for a simple two-period two-group crossover study is

	period 1		period 2	
	treatment	mean effect	treatment	mean effect
Group 1 (n_1) 1	1	$y_{1.1}$	2	$y_{1.2}$
Group 2 (n_2) 2	2	$y_{2.1}$	1	$y_{2..2}$

where y_{ijk} = the response in the jth patient in the ith group in the kth period. We assume that $n_1 = n_2 = n$ and that we have normal distributions or t-distributions. $y_{i.k} = \Sigma y_{ijk}/n$.

Treatment, carryover and time effects are assessed according to Grizzle.[11] To test treatment effect φ the sum of the results of treatment 1 is compared with the treatment 2 results ($y_{1.1}+y_{2.2}$ vs $y_{1.2}+y_{2.1}$). To trace carryover effect(λ) the sum of the results in group 1 is compared with the group 2 results($y_{1.1}+y_{1.2}$ vs $y_{2.1}+y_{2.2}$). To trace time effect(π) the sum of the results in period 1 is compared with the period 2 results($y_{1.1}+y_{2.1}$ vs $y_{1.2}+y_{2.2}$).

The null-hypotheses that φ, λ, and π are zero

.
$$\varphi \quad [(y_{1.1}+y_{2.2})-(y_{1.2}+y_{2.1})]=0$$
.
$$\lambda \quad [(y_{2.1}+y_{2.2})-(y_{1.1}+y_{1.2})]=0$$
.
$$\pi \quad [(y_{1.1}+y_{2.1})-(y_{1.2}+y_{2.2})]=0$$

should be slightly remodeled into paired comparisons, because otherwise calculations cannot be appropriately accomplished.

.
$$\varphi \quad [(y_{1.1}-y_{1.2})-(y_{2.1}-y_{2.2})]=0$$
.
$$\lambda \quad [(y_{2.1}+y_{2.2})-(y_{1.1}+y_{1.2})]=0$$
.
$$\pi \quad [(y_{1.1}-y_{1.2})+(y_{2.1}-y_{2.2})]=0$$

In this way 2x2 paired cells can be adequately added or subtracted in a cell by cell manner.

4. HYPOTHESIS TESTING

These null hypotheses can be tested, for example, by paired t-statistic or repeated measures analysis of variance(ANOVA). The larger the extent to which the t or F value of our distribution differs from zero, the more sensitivity the statistical approach does provide.

$$t = \frac{d}{SE} \quad \text{(or repeated measures ANOVA,F value)}$$

where d is φ, λ, or π, and SE is their standard error.
SE is calculated by use of the standard formulas for the variance ($\sqrt{\sigma^2/n}$) of paired and unpaired sums and differences.

.
$$\sigma^2_{paired\ sums} = \sigma_1^2 + \sigma_2^2 + 2\rho\,\sigma_1\sigma_2$$
.
$$\sigma^2_{paired\ differences} = \sigma_1^2 + \sigma_2^2 - 2\rho\,\sigma_1\sigma_2$$
.
$$\sigma^2_{unpaired\ sums} = \sigma_1^2 + \sigma_2^2$$
.
$$\sigma^2_{unpaired\ differences} = \sigma_1^2 + \sigma_2^2$$

If we assume that $\sigma = \sigma_{Y1.1} = \sigma_{Y1.2} = \sigma_{Y2.1} = \sigma_{Y2.2}$= standard deviation of the samples in each of the cells, and that $\rho = \rho_{Y1.1\ vs\ Y1.2} = \rho_{Y2.1\ vs\ Y2.2}$ = correlation coefficient between the samples of each of the two paired cells, then

.
$$\sigma_\varphi^2 = 2(2\sigma^2)(1-\rho)$$
.
$$\sigma_\lambda^2 = 2(2\sigma^2)(1+\rho)$$
.
$$\sigma_\pi^2 = 2(2\sigma^2)(1-\rho)$$

Because $n_1 = n_2 = n$, we now can calculate the SEs as follows:

$$SE_{\varphi_-} = \sqrt{4\sigma^2(1-\rho)(1/2n + 1/2n)}$$
$$= \sqrt{4\sigma^2(1-\rho)/n}$$

and accordingly

$$SE_\lambda = \sqrt{4\sigma^2(1+\rho)/n}$$
$$SE_\pi = \sqrt{4\sigma^2(1-\rho)/n}$$

Suppose $\lambda=\varphi$ and $\rho= 0$, then $t_\lambda = t_\varphi$. In this situation the sensitivity to test carryover and treatment effect are equal.

If $\lambda=\varphi$ and $\rho > 0$ then $t_\lambda < t_\varphi$
If $\lambda=\varphi$ and $\rho < 0$ then $t_\lambda > t_\varphi$

So, the sensitivity of testing is largely dependent on the correlation between treatment modalities ρ. Whenever $\rho > 0$ we soon will have a much larger t, and , thus, better sensitivity to test treatment effect than carryover effect of similar size. We should add that in practice $\sigma_{Y1.2}$ may be somwhat larger than $\sigma_{Y1.1}$, because the larger the data the larger the variances. If, e.g., $\sigma_{Y1.2}$ is 10% larger than $\sigma_{Y1.1}$, ρ will change from 0.00 to 0.05. So, in this situation the level of positive correlation required tends to rise.

Time effect(π) is generally considered to influence one treatment similarly to the other, and its influence on the size of the treatment difference is, thus, negligible.

	Treatment	Period 1 Mean response	Period 2 Treatment	Mean response
Group 1	1	$y_{1.1}$	2	$y_{1.2}+\tfrac{1}{2}\pi$
Group 2	2	$y_{2.1}$	1	$y_{2.2}+\tfrac{1}{2}\pi$

Under the assumption $\varphi = 0$ we have
$$\varphi = (y_{1.1}-y_{1.2}-\tfrac{1}{2}\pi)-(y_{2.1}-y_{2.2}-\tfrac{1}{2}\pi)$$
$$= y_{1.1}-y_{1.2}-y_{2.1}+y_{2.2}$$

Although time or period effects may introduce extra variance in the study, the crossover design in a way adjusts for time effects, and some even believe that time effects do not have to be taken into account in the routine analysis of crossover studies, unless there is a clinical interest to know.[7]

5. STATISTICAL POWER OF TESTING

PROBABILITY
DISTRIBUTION

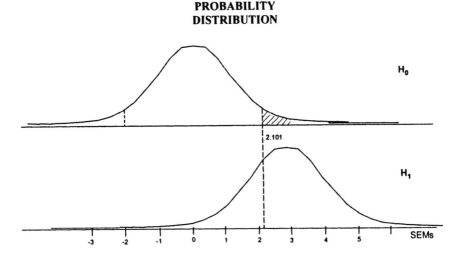

Fig. 1.Example of a t-distribution (H₁) and its null hypothesis (H₀).

Fig. 1.Example of a t-distribution (H_1) and its null hypothesis (H_0).
α = % chance of erroneously rejecting this null hypothesis (usually taken as 5%), β=
% chance of erroneously accepting this null hypothesis. Statistical power is defined as
$(1-\beta)x$ 100%.

Figure 1 gives an example of a t-distribution (H_1)and its null hypothesis of no effect (H_0). α = % chance of erroneously rejecting this null hypothesis (usually taken as 5%), and β=% chance of erroneously accepting this null hypothesis. Statistical power is defined as $(1-\beta)$ x 100%. Statistical power can be approximated from the equation

$$POWER = 1 - \beta = 1 - prob\ [Z \le (t^1 - t)]$$

where Z represents the standardized value for the differences between mean and zero and t^1 represents the upper critical value of t for the given degrees of freedom and α has been specified (α = 0.05).

Suppose we have a crossover study with n=10 per group, because this is a size frequently used in such studies, and with $\varphi = \sigma$ = standard deviation of the samples in each cell, because this is frequently approximately so. Then increasing amounts of λ are added with σ_λ = . The influence of this procedure on the statistical power of testing λ and φ are then assessed. The amounts of λ are expressed as λ/φ ratios. Power graphs are calculated for three different levels of correlation-between-drug-response ($\rho \cong -1$; $\rho \cong 0$; $\rho \cong +1$).

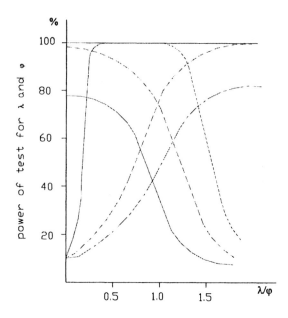

Fig . 2. Statistical power of testing carryover effect (slope upwards) and
treatment effect (slope downwards); λ= carryover effect, φ= treatment
effect, ρ = correlation coefficient.

$$\rule{4cm}{0.4pt} \quad \rho \cong -1$$
$$- - - - - - - \quad \rho \cong 0$$
$$\text{-------------------} \quad \rho \cong +1$$

Figure 2 shows the results. First, there are three power curves of treatment effect for
the three levels of correlation. As λ/φ increases, all three gradually come down. The
negative correlation curve is the first to do so. Consequently, this situation has
generally little power of rightly coming to the right conclusion. At λ/φ= 1.0 , when
treatment effect is equal to carryover effect, there is less than 30% power left. It
means we have a more than 70% chance that treatment effect is erroneously
unobserved in this study. Considering that a power of approximately 80% is
required for reliable testing, we cannot test carryover here in a sensitive manner.
The zero and positive correlation situations provide essentially better power.
There are also three power curves of carryover effect for three correlation levels.
The negative correlation curve provides essentially better power than the zero and
positive correlation curves do. This example shows that strong positive correlations
leave little power to test carryover effect.It also shows that strong negative
correlations produce excessive power to test carryover effect.
The amounts of time effect is generally assumed to influence the two treatment
groups similarly, and it, therefore, may hardly influence the treat comparison.
Suppose in the above example time effect (π) instead of carryover effect (λ) is
added in increasing amounts with σ_π=π.

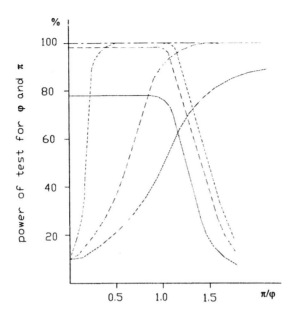

Fig. 3. Statistical power of testing time effect (slope upwards) and treatment effect (slope downwards). π= time effect, φ= treatment effect, ρ= correlation coefficient.

_____ $\rho \cong -1$

_ _ _ _ _ _ _ _ $\rho \cong 0$

- - - - - - - - - - - - - $\rho \cong +1$

Figure 3 shows the influence of increasing ratios π/φ on the statistical power of testing π and φ. First, small time effects unlike carryover effects hardly influence nor the amount nor the statistical power of testing treatment effect. Also the power of demonstrating time effect is largely dependent on the level of correlation-between-drug-response: with a negative correlation we have little power to demonstrate time-effect. In contrast, with a positive correlation we have a lot of power to do so.

We conclude that the level of correlation-between-drug-reponse is a major determinant of not only the power of demonstrating treatment effect but also that of time effect in the current approach.

6. CONCLUSIONS

The crossover design for treatment comparisons with continuous variables provides approximately equal statistical power to test carryover, time, and treatment effects when between-treatment correlation is not strong positive/negative. E.g., in the hypothesized crossover situation from our example the statistical power to demonstrate similarly-sized treatment and carryover, or treatment and time effects is approximately 80% (as demonstrated in the above figures), which is generally considered to be an acceptable level for reliable testing. However, whenever the correlation coefficient is >0, we will soon have better sensitivity to test treatment than carryover or time effect of similar size. Inversely, whenever it is <0, we will soon have better sensitivity to demonstrate the latter two rather than the former.

We should add that calculations are made under the assumption that either carryover or time effect are in the study. If both effects are simultaneously in the study, variances have to be added up and powers will be somewhat smaller. The assumption does not invalidate the overall conclusion of the procedure as it produces the largest powers for the given data.

ANCOVA (ANALYSIS OF COVARIANCE)

When F-tests are used instead of t-tests, the sensitivity of testing can be simply adjusted by analysis of covariance (ANCOVA) according to

$$\text{adjusted } SS_{treatment} \text{ between groups} =$$
$$\text{unadjusted } SS_{treatment} \text{ between groups} +$$
$$(SP \text{ within groups})^2/SS_{carryover} \text{ within groups} -$$
$$(SP \text{ total})^2/SS_{carryover} \text{ total}$$

$$\text{adjusted } SS \text{ within groups} = \text{unadjusted } SS \text{ within groups} -$$
$$(SP \text{ within groups})^2/SS_{carryover} \text{ within groups}$$

where SS= sum of squares, and SP= sum of products of
treatment by carryover effects
(treatment effect x carryover effect).

Computation can be found, e.g., in Hays' textbook Statistics[12],and can be readily made by statistical packages, e.g., SPSS[13] under the subprogram "ANOVA".

In this way, power of testing may improve by a few percentages. However, this method of adjustment can be used only when corrrelations are not strong + or - , and when n is not at least 20 or more, which is not so in many crossover studies. Also the method only adjusts statistical sensitivity, but not amounts of treatment, carryover or time effects, and so its usefullness is limited.

Although the analysis uses multiple comparison testing, the p values do not have to be multiplied by the number of tests, because although the chance of a positive test increases, the chance of e.g., a positive test for carryover does not as it is only tested once.

The current chapter stresses the major impact of correlation level between treatment comparison, and particularly the phenomenon of negative correlations. This phenomenon is only shortly being recognized and may have flawed many trials so far. In a trial the test treatment is frequently a slight modification of the reference treatment or is equivalent to it with addition of just a new component. In this situation there is obviously a positive correlation between responses to test and reference treatments. However, completely new classes of drugs are continually being developed and are tested against established classes of drugs. With the comparison of drugs from completely different classes patients may fall into different populations: those who respond better to one class and those who do so to the other class.. E.g., patients with angina pectoris unresponsive to calcium channel blockers or nitrates. may respond very well to beta blockers. Also hypertension, cardiac arrhythmias, chronic obstructive pulmonary disease are conditions where a non-response is frequently associated with an excellent response to a completely different compound. These are situations where a crosssover study may give rise to a strong negative correlation. It would mean that a crossover design for the comparisons of treatment from completely different classes of drugs is endangered of being flawed and that such comparisons had better be assessed in the form of a parallel group comparison which evens out within subject variability.

7. REFERENCES

1. Niemeyer MG, Zwinderman AH, Cleophas TJ, De Vogel EM. Crossover studies are a better format for comparing equivalent treatments than parallel-group studies. In: Kuhlmann J, Mrozikiewicz A, eds, What should a clinical pharmacologist know to start a clinical trial (phase I and II). Munich, Germany, Zuckschwerdt Verlag, 1998, pp 40-8.
2. Scheffé H. Mixed models. In: Scheffé H, ed, The analysis of variance. New York, Wiley & Sons, 1959, pp 261-91.
3. Cleophas TJ. Crossover studies: a modified analysis with more power. Clin Pharmacol Ther 1993; 53: 515-20.
4. Willan AR,Pater JL. Carryover and the two-period crossover clinical trial . Biometrics 1986; 42: 593-9.
5. Freeman PR. The performance of the two-stage analysis of two-treatment, two-period crossover trials . Stat Med 1989; 8: 1421-32.
6. Fleiss JA. A critique of recent research on the two-treatment crossover design . Control Clin Trials 1989; 10: 237-41.
7. Senn S. The AB/BA crosover: past, present and future. Stat Methods Med Res 1994; 3: 303-24.
8. Grieve AP. Bayesian analyses of two-treatment crossover studies. Stat Methods Med Res 1994; 3: 407-29.

9.Cleophas TJ, Van Lier HH. Clinical trials with binary responses: power analyses. J Clin Pharmacol 1996; 36: 198-204.

10.Nies AS, Spielberg SP. Individualization of drug therapy. In: Hardman JL et al., eds, Goodman and Gilman's Pharmacological Basis of Therapeutics . New York: McGraw-Hill,1996, pp 43-63.

11.Grizzle JE. The two-period change-over design and its use in clinical trials. Bbiometrics 1965; 22: 469-80.

12.SPSS 8 for Windows 95 and 98, SPSS Benelux, Gorinchem, Netherlands.

13.Hays WL. Statistics. Fort Worth, TX, Holt, Rinehart and Winston, Inc, 4th edition, 1991.

CHAPTER 13

CROSSOVER STUDIES WITH BINARY RESPONSES

1. SUMMARY

The two-period crossover trial has the evident advantage that by the use of within-patients comparisons, the usually larger between-patient variability is not used as a measuring stick to compare treatments. However, a prerequisite is that the order of the treatments does not substantially influence the outcome of the treatment. Crossover studies with a binary response (such as yes/no or present/absent), although widely used for initial screening of new compounds, have not previously been studied for such order effects. In the present paper we use a mathematical model based on standard statistical tests to study to what extent such order effects, here identical to carryover effects, may reduce the power of detecting a treatment effect. We come to the conclusion that in spite of large carryover effects the crossover study with a binary response remains a powerful method and that testing for carryover effects makes sense only if the null hypothesis of no treatment effect cannot be rejected.

2. INTRODUCTION

The crossover design is widely used in clinical research especially in the case of a limited number of patients. The main advantage of within-patient over between-patient comparisons is that between-subject variability is not used in the comparisons. However, a prerequisite is that the order of the treatments does not influence the outcome of the treatment. If the effect of the treatment administered in the 1st period carries on into the 2nd period then it may influence the measured response in the 2nd period. This essentially means that only symptomatic treatments qualify for crossover comparisons and curative treatments do not. However, symptomatic treatments frequently have small curative effects, e.g., wound healing by vasodilators or, more recently, cardiac remodelling by afterload reduction. The treatment group that is treated with the effective compound first and with the less effective compound or placebo second is frequently biased by carryover effect from the 1st period into the 2nd, whereas the alternative group that is treated in the reverse order is not so [1]. For example, of 73 recently published crossovers only 6 reported the data of the separate periods. In 5 of them (83%) this very type of carryover effect was demonstrable. Such a mechanism may cause a severe underestimation of the treatment results[2] and this possibility should, therefore, be assessed in the analysis. Most of the reports on the subject of order effects so far have addressed crossover studies with a quantitative rather than binary response [3-10]. Although Hills & Armitage [11] in an overview of methods in crossover clinical trials mentioned the tests of Gart [12] and Prescott[13] for crossover trials with a binary response and Fidler [14] presented a model, little attention has been paid to this kind of trials. A binary respons is different from a quantitative in that it generally does not answer what exactly can be expected in an individual. Rather it addresses whether or not a particular result has a predictive value, which one of two treatments is better, or whether there is a treatment effect in the data. One might contend, therefore, that some undervaluation of a difference in binary data is not that important as long as it does not cause a type II error of finding no difference were there is one. The main issue of the present paper is the question whether in a crossover trial with a binary response a significant carryover effect does leave enough power in the data to demonstrate a treatment effect.

3. ASSESSMENT OF CARRYOVER AND TREATMENT EFFECT

In a crossover trial with two treatments and two periods the patients are randomized into two symmetric groups that are treated with treatments A and B in a different order (table 1). If groups are symmetric and the results are not influenced by the order of the treatments the probabilities of treatment success in group I and II should be virtually the same in each period for each treatment: p_A being the probability of treatment success from treatment A, p_B from treatment B (table 1).

Table 1. Example of a crossover design with a binary response

		Period 1			Period II
	Treatment	Probability of treatment success		Treatment	Probility of treatment success
Group I	A	p_A		B	p_B
Group II	B	p_B		A	p_A*

* If in Group II treatment B has a carryover effect on the outcome of treatment A, p_A changes to p_C. If $P_B = p_C$, carryover effect is maximal.

The group that is treated with the less effective treatment or placebo after the more effective is endangered of being biased by carryover effect from the 1st period into the 2nd.

Suppose treatment A is far less effective than B (table 1). Then, if in Group II treatment B has a carryover effect on the outcome of treatment A, the probability of treatment success changes from p_B into p_C. To detect a carryover effect we compare the outcomes of treatment A in Group I to those in group II: p_A versus p_C, an unpaired comparison. The amount of carryover effect in group II is considered to be the difference between p_C and p_A. Carryover effect in Group I (ineffective treatment period prior to effective) is assumed to be negligible. Time effect is assumed to be negligible as well because we study stable disease only. It thus seems that neither a test for carryover effect in Group I, nor a test for time effects needs to be included in our assessment. Treatment effect is assessed by taking the two groups together after which all of the outcomes of the treatments A are compared with those of the treatments B in a paired comparison. The assumption that carryover effect is negligible implies that the test for carryover effect uses only half of the available data and might therefore be expected to be less sensitive. However, sensitivity not only depends on sample size but also on the size of differences and their variances.

4. STATISTICAL MODEL FOR TESTING TREATMENT AND CARRYOVER EFFECTS

We assume an unidirectional assessment where p is between 0.0 (no symptoms anymore) and 1.0 (=100% remains symptomatic in spite of treatment). When carryover effect is in the data, p_A in Group II turns into p_C (table 1). The difference between p_C and p_A is considered to be the amount of carryover effect in the data. Fisher exact test, as explained in chapter 3, is used for testing whether p_C is significantly different from p_A. With the program of Bavry [15] those values of p_C are determined that should yield a significant carryover effect in 80% of the trials (i.e. the power equals 80%). The number of patients in both groups is chosen between 10 and 25, because many crossover trials have 20 to 50 patients. These values of p_C are then used for determining whether in crossover trials with significant carryover effect and a binary response enough power is left in the data for demonstrating a significant treatment effect.

For testing the treatment effect all of the data of the treatment A are for that purpose taken together and compared with those of the treatments B. The power of this test depends not only on the probabilities p_A and p_B, but also on the correlation between the treatment responses. This correlation is expressed as $\rho = p_{A/B} - p_A$, where $p_{A/B}$ is the probability of a treatment success with A, given that treatment B was successful. When $\rho = 0$ treatments A and B act independently. When p_B equals p_C, this would mean that carryover effect in group II is not only significant but also maximal given the amount of treatment effect. Considering this situation of maximal carryover effect, we calculate the power of detecting treatment effects. The power of McNemar test with p_B being equal to p_C and various values for was calculated according to Bavry [15].

5. RESULTS

CALCULATION OF PC VALUES JUST YIELDING A SIGNIFICANT TEST FOR CARRYOVER EFFECT

For various numbers of patients and various values of p_A (the probability of success with treatment A in period I, table 1), the p_C values (the probability of success with treatment A in period II) are calculated that with a power of 80% will give a significant test for carryover effect (p_A vs P_C, $\alpha = 0.05$).

Table 2 shows that carryover effects (difference between p_A and p_C) as large as 0.60, 0.50, 0.40 and 0.35 are required for a significant test. For $\alpha = 0.01$, these values are about 0.70, 0.60, 0.50 and 0.45. Using these p_C values, we then calculated the probability of detecting a treatment effect (i.e. power of testing treatment effect). We report minimal values of power only, i.e., the situation where $p_B = p_C$. Whenever $p_B < p_C$, we would have even better power of testing treatment effect.

Table 2. Power to demonstrate a treatment effect in spite of the presence of a significant carryover effect

	Total number of patients			
p_A	2 x 10	2 x 15	2 x 20	2 x 25
0.10				
0.20				
0.30				98(0.02)
0.40		96(0.02)	97(0.05)	96(0.08)
0.50		97(0.06)	96(0.11)	96(0.14)
0.60	97*(0.04)#	98(0.11)	96(0.18)	95(0.23)
0.70	96(0.11)	97(0.20)	97(0.26)	94(0.33)
0.80	96(0.20)	97(0.30)	97(0.37)	96(0.43)
0.90	96(0.31)	97(0.43)	96(0.47)	96(0.52)

* Power (%) of McNemar test for treatment effect ($\alpha = 0.05$, $\rho = 0$).
# p_C value just yielding a significant test for carryover effect ($\alpha = 0.05$, power = 80%).

POWER OF PAIRED COMPARISON FOR TREATMENT EFFECT

When the result of treatment B (p_B) is taken equal to the maximal values of p_C and treatments A and B act independently ($\rho = 0$), the probability of detecting a treatment effect (i.e. the power) in the crossover situation with n between 20 and 50 is always more than 94% (ttable 2). Usually, however, treatments A and B do not act independently. With a negative correlation between the two treatments modalities power is lost, with a positive correlation it is augmented. Table 3 shows power values adjusted for different levels of ρ. With negative levels of ρ and 20 patients the power for detecting a treatment difference is not less than 74% which is about as large as that chosen for the test on carryover effect (80%). When more patients are admitted to the trial this value will be about 90%.

Table 3. Power (%) to demonstrate a treatment effect in spite of the presence of a significant carryover effect

| | ρ | Total number of patients | | | |
		2 x 10	2 x 15	2 x 20	2 x 25
$\alpha_1^* = 0.05$	-0.20	89	94	96	95
$\alpha_2 = 0.05$	-0.10	92	96	97	97
	0	96	96	96	94
	0.10	98	97	98	99
	0.20	98	98	99	99
$\alpha_1 = 0.01$	-0.20	95	99	94	99
$\alpha_2 = 0.01$	-0.10	97	100	99	99
	0	99	99	99	99
	0.10	100	100	100	100
	0.20	100	100	100	100
$\alpha_1 = 0.10$	-0.20	74	84	89	88
$\alpha_2 = 0.05$	-0.10	79	91	92	90
	0	85	90	89	88
	0.10	89	95	95	94
	0.20	95	94	97	97
$\alpha_1 = 0.05$	-0.20	75	87	90	90
$\alpha_2 = 0.01$	-0.10	81	92	92	93
	0	88	90	90	89
	0.10	92	93	95	96
	0.20	96	96	98	98

* α_1 level of significance of test for carryover effect.
α_2 level of significance of test for treatment effect.
ρ level of correlation between treatments A and B.

6. EXAMPLES

Suppose we have a negative crossover where probability of treatment success group II p_C (Table IV) may have changed from 0.8 into 0.2 due to carryover effect from the effective treatment B into the 2nd period. Fisher exact test for demonstrating a carryover effect (p_A vs p_C) is calculated according to

Point probability for
carryover effect $= \dfrac{10! \; 10! \; 10! \; 10!}{20! \; 2! \; 8! \; 2! \; 8!} = 0.011$

Cumulative tail probability = 0.011 + 0.003 + 0.007 = 0.021 and is thus significant at an $\alpha = 0.021$ level.

If we perform a similar unpaired analysis of the first period for demonstrating a treatment effect we likewise obtain a significant test at $\alpha = 0.021$ level. Suppose carryover effect would be smaller, e.g., $p_A = 0.8$, $p_B = 0.0$, $p_C = 0.2$. Then the test for treatment effect would yield an even better result:

Point probability for
carryover effect $= \dfrac{29! \; 8! \; 10! \; 10!}{20! \; 2! \; 8! \; 10! \; 0!} = 0.004$

Cumulative tail probability = 0.004 + 0.001 + 0.003 = 0.008.

So, in crossovers with a binary response and a negative result, it does make sense to test for carryover effect by comparing the two periods with the less effective treatment modalities. If a significant test is demonstrated, we obviously will find a significant difference at a similar or even lower level of significance when taking the 1st period for estimating the difference between treatment A and B. Thus, it would seem appropriate for our purpose to disregard the data of the 2nd period in this particular situation (although the 2nd period might still provide interesting information).

Table 4. Example

		Period I		Period II	
	Treatment	Probability of treatment success		Treatment	Probability of treatment success
Group I (n=10)	A	$p_A = 0.8$		B	$p_B = 0.2$
Group II (n=10)	B	$p_B = 0.2$		A	$p_C = 0.2$

7. DISCUSSION

The power of crossover studies is frequently reduced by carryover effect. This is particularly so when a group that is treated with an effective treatment first, is then treated with an ineffective treatment or placebo second. In studies with a quantitative response this very effect may cause severe underestimation of the treatment effect [1]. Studies with a binary response are, however, different from studies with a quantitative response in that they are mostly designed to answer whether a treatment has any effect rather than what size such effect does have. One might contend, therefore, that underestimation in such studies is not that important as long as the null hypothesis of no treatment effect doesn't have to be erroneously accepted. We demonstrate that in crossovers with a binary response and significant carryover effect the power of testing the treatment effect remains substantial even so. This would imply that routinely testing for carryover effects in such studies is not necessary as long as the result of the treatment comparison is positive. When a study is negative it does make sense, however, to test for carryover effect by comparing p_A vs p_C (Table I).

When p_A is significantly different from p_C, we assume that there is carryover effect in group II. In this situation a parallel-group analysis of period I (p_A vs p_B) can effectively be used for the purpose of demonstrating a treatment effect. It will provide a significant difference at the same or even a lower level of significance than the test for carryover effect. This is so, because when carryover effect is maximal, p_B equals p_C. The difference between p_B and p_A will, therefore, be at least as large as the difference between p_C and p_A but probably larger. Therefore, no further test for treatment effect seems to be required for our purpose and it seems appropriate that the results of the 2nd period be disregarded.

Considering that the problem of carryover effects influence in crossover trials with a binary response may not be too hard to handle, we may as well shift our standard of choosing this particular trial design somewhat, and make use of its additional advantages more frequently. The design is, e.g., particularly powerful for the study of rapid relief of symptoms in chronic disease where the long-term condition of the patient remains fairly stable [16]. This is so, because between-subject variability is not used in a within-subject comparison. Also, we can make use of positive correlations between the treatment modalities tested, because the statistical power of testing treatment comparisons with a positive correlation can be largely enhanced by within-subject comparisons [17]. Furthermore, none of the patients in the trial has to be treated throughout the trial with a less adequate dose or placebo, which is why a crossover raises usually less ethical problems than does a parallel-group study where one group is treated with a placebo or less adequate dosage throughout the trial. Also, we have the advantage that patients can express their own opinions about which of the treatments they personally prefer. This is especially important with subjective variables, such as pain scores.

Furthermore, not so large a group is required because of within-subject comparisons, which facilitates the recruitment procedure and reduces costs. Finally, double-blinding cannot be effectively executed in selfcontrolled studies without some kind of crossover design.

CONCLUSSIONS

1. Crossover studies with a binary response and positive results do not have to be tested for carryover effects.
2. If such studies have a negative result, testing for carryover effect does make sense.
3. If a carryover effect is demonstrated the treatment results should be analyzed in the form of a parallel-group study of the 1st period.

8. REFERENCES

1. Cleophas TJM: A simple analysis of carryover studies with one-group interaction. Int J Clin Pharmacol Ther 1995; 32: 322-8.
2. Cleophas TJ: Underestimation of treatment effect in crossover trials. Angiology 1990; 41: 855-64.
3. Brown BW: The crossover experiment for clinical trials.Biometrics 1980;36:69-79
4. Barker M, Hew RJ, Huitson A, Poloniecki J: The two-period crossover trial. Bias 1982; 9: 67-112.
5. Louis TA, Lavori PW, Bailar JC, Polansky M: Crossover and self-controlled design in clinical research. N Engl J Med 1984; 310: 24-31.
6. Willan AR, Pater JL: Carryover and the two-period clinical trial. Biometrics 1986; 42: 593-9.
7. Packer M: Combined beta-adrenergic and calcium entry blockade in angina pectoris. N Engl J Med 1989; 320: 709-18.
8. Fleiss JL: A critique of recent research on the two-treatment crossover design. Control Clin Trials 1989; 10: 237-43.
9. Freeman PR: The performance of the two-stage analysis of two-treatment, two-period crossover trials. Stat Med 1989; 8: 1421-32.
10. Senn S. Crossover trials in clinical research. Wiley & Sons, Chicester, 1993.
11. Hills M. Armitage P: The two-period crossover trial. Br J Clin Pharmacol 1979; 8: 7-20.
12. Gart JJ: An exact test for comparing matched proportions in crossover designs. Biometrika 1969; 56: 57-80.
13. Prescott RJ: The comparison of success rates in crossover trials in the presence of an order effect. Appl Stat 1981; 30: 9-15.
14. Fidler V: Change-over clinical trials with binary data: mixed model-based comparisons of tests. Biometrics 1984; 40: 1063-79.
15. Bavry JH: Design Power (TM). Scientific software Inc., 1988, Hillsdale, New Jersey.
16. Cleophas TJM, Tavenier P. Clinical trials of chronic diseases. J Clin Pharmacol 1995; 35: 594-8.
17. Cleophas TJM, Tavenier P. Fundamental issues of choosing the right type of trial. Am J Ther 1994; 1: 327-32.

CHAPTER 14

POST-HOC ANALYSIS IN CLINICAL TRIALS, A CASE FOR LOGISTIC REGRESSION ANALYSIS

1. MULTIVARIATE METHODS

Multivariate methods are used to adjust asymmetries in the patient characteristics in a trial. It can also be used for a subsequent purpose. In many trials simple primary hypotheses in terms of efficacy and safety expectations, are tested through their respective outcome variables as described in the protocol. However, sometimes it is decided already at the design stage that post hoc analyses will be performed for the purpose of testing secondary hypotheses. E.g., suppose we first want to know whether a novel beta-blocker is better than a standard beta-blocker, and second, if so, whether this better effect is due to a vasodilatory property of the novel compound. The first hypothesis is assessed in the primary (univariate) analysis. For the second hypothesis, we can simply adjust the two treatment groups for difference in vasodilation by multiple regression analysis and see whether differences in treatment effects otherwise are affected by this procedure. However, with small data power is lost by such procedure. More power is provided by the following approach. We could assign all of the patients to two new groups: patients who actually have improvement in the primary outcome variable and those who have not, irrespective of the type of beta-blocker. We, then, can perform a regression analyis of the two new groups trying to find independent determinants of this improvement. If one or more determinants for adjustment are binary, which is generally so, our choice of test is logistic regression analysis. Testing the second hypothesis is, of course, of lower validity than testing the first one, because it is post-hoc and makes use of a regression analysis which does not differentiate between causal relationships and relationships due to an unknown common factor.

2. EXAMPLES

In a double-blind randomized study of the new beta-blocker celiprolol for patients with angina pectoris the main outcome variable was anginal attack rate. Additional outcome variables include systolic and diastolic blood pressure, heart rate, rate pressure product, peripheral vascular resistance. Although this study measures several outcomes, the various outcomes to some degree measure the same thing, and this may be particularly so with blood pressure, heart rate and pressure rate product since they are assumed to represent oxygen demand to the heart, which is jeopardized during anginal attacks. The new beta-blocker has been demonstrated preclinically not only to reduce rate pressure product like any other beta-blocker but also to reduce peripheral vascular resistance. The novel beta-blocker indeed performed significantly better than the latter (persistent angina pectoris at the completion of the trial 17 versus 33 %, P<0.01, 1-β= ±80%), and this was accompanied by a significantly better reduction of systolic blood pressure and reduction of peripheral resistance. A problem with multivariate analysis is its relatively small power with usual sample sizes. For the purpose of better power patients may be divided into new groups according to their main outcome. In order to determine the most important determinants of the better clinical benefit, the patients were therefore divided into two new groups: they were assigned to "no-angina-pectoris"at the completion of the trial or "persistent-angina-pectoris"(Table I). Univariate analysis of these two new groups showed that most of the

Table 1.Angina pectoris and odds ratios of persistent angina pectoris in the celiprolol (novel compound) and propranolol (reference compound) group adjusted for independent variables (data from Cleophas et al; Clin Pharmacol Ther 1996;45: 476). Odds ratio= occurrence rate ratio of persistent angina pectoris celiprolol group/occcurrence rate ratio of persistent angina pectoris propranolol group. Means ±SDs are given

	No angina pectoris (n=23)	P	persistent angina pectoris (n=30)
systolic blood pressure(mm Hg)	134± 17	<0.001	155± 19
diastolic blood pressure (mm Hg)	77± 13	<0.02	84± 9
heart rate (beat/min)	65 ± 9	<0.09	69± 9
rate pressure product (mm Hg.Beats/min.10^{-3})	8.6±11	<0.001	10.7±14
fore arm blood flow (ml/100ml tissue.min)	8.8±10.8	<0.02	4.1±2.2
treatment assignment (celiprolol/propanolol)	18/5	<0.001	8/22

	odds ratio of persistent angina	95% CIs	P-value
unadjusted	0.38	0.25-0.52	<0.002
adjusted for rate pressure product	0.13	0.05-0.22	<0.0005
adjusted for systolic pressure plus heart rate	0.12	0.04-0.20	<0.0005

additional outcome variables including treatment assignment were significantly different between the two groups. These variables were entered in the logistic regression analysis: the variables double product, systolic blood pressure and heart rate were independent of treatment assignment, while peripheral flow (=1/peripheral vascular resistance) was not. After adjustment for flow the difference in treatment asssignment was lost. This suggests that celiprolol exerted its beneficial effect to a large extent through its peripheral vasodilatory property.

A double-blind randomized parallel-group study compared chronotropic (mibefradil ands diltiazem) and non-chronotropic calcium channel blockers (amlodipine) in patients with angina pectoris. Although all of the calcium channel blockers improved exercise tolerance as estimated by % increased time to onset ischemia during bicycle ergometry, mibefradil and diltiazem performed better than amlodipine (20.8 and 12.4 s versus 9.9 s, P<0.01 and < 0.001). In order to determine the most important determinants of this better clinical benefit, patients were divided into two new groups: they were assigned to non-responders if their change in ischemic onset time was zero or less, and to responders if it was larger than zero (Table II). Univariate analysis of these two groups showed that many variables including treatment assignment were significantly different between the two groups.

Table 2. Mean data (SDs) after assignment of patients according to whether (responders) or not (non-responders) their ischemia-onset-time increased after treatment with calcium channel blockers , and odds ratios of mibefradil or diltiazem versus amlodipine for responding, unadjusted and after adjustment for difference of heart rate (Cleophas et al; Br J Clin Pharmacol 1999; 50: 545). Odds ratio=occurrence rate ratio responders on mibefradil or diltiazem or amlodipine / occurrence rate ratio on amlodipine

	responders (n=239)	non-responders (n=61)	P-value
at rest			
systolic blood pressure (mm Hg)	−5 (19)	-1 (23)	0.27
diastolic blood pressure (mm Hg)	- 5 (10)	-3 (10)	0.13 heart
rate (beats/min)	-5 (11.0)	1.1 (9.6)	<0.001
rate pressure product			
(mm Hg.beats/min.10^{-3})	−1.0(1.9)	0.1 (2.1)	<0.001
at maximal workload			
systolic blood pressure (mm Hg)	-1(21)	-2 (27)	0.68
diastolic blood pressure (mm Hg)	-4(11)	-4(11)	0.97
heart rate (beats/min)	-12(17)	-6(15)	0.010
rate pressure product			
(mm Hg.beats/min.10^{-3})	-2.3(4.5)	−1.2 (4.5)	0.090
treatment assignment(n %)			
amlodipine	76(32%)	27(44%)	
diltiazem	75(31%)	26(43%)	
mibefradil	88(37%)	8(13%)	

	raw odds ratio (95% CIs)	odds ratio adjusted for change in heart rate (95% CIs)
amlodipine	1 (-)	1(-)
diltiazem	1.02 (0.55-1.92)	0.86 (0.45-1.66)
mibefradil	3.91 (1.68-9.11)	2.26 (0.86-5.97)

These variables were entered into the logistic regression analysis: the difference in treatment assignment between the two groups was lost after adjustment for heart rates. This suggests that the beneficial effect of calcium channel blockers in this category of patients is largely dependent upon their effect on heart rate.

It is important to recognize that in the first study there is a positive correlation between peripheral flow and clinical benefit (when peripheral flow increases benefit gets better), whereas in the second study there is a negative correlation between heart rate and clinical benefit(when heart increases benefit gets worse). Multivariate analysis only measures dependencies but makes no differences between a positive and negative correlation. So, we must not forget to look at the trend in the data before interpretations can be made.

3. LOGISTIC REGRESSION EQUATION

Logistic regression is similar to linear regression of which main equation as explained in chapter 8 is

$$y = a + b_1 x_1 + b_2 x_2 + \ldots b_n x_n$$

Linear regression software finds for you an equation that best predicts the outcome y from one or more x variables. Continuous data are measured. Y is assumed to be the expected value of a normal distribution. With y being a binary (yes/no) variable, the proportion of, e.g., yes data (p) lies between 0 and 1, and this is too small a range of values for the expression of a summary of multiple variables like $a + b_1 x_1 + b_2 x_2 + \ldots b_n x_n$. The range of y-responses can be broadened to 0 to ∞ if we take $p(1-p)$ as y-variable , and even to $-\infty$ to $+\infty$ if we take $\ln p(1-p)$. The simplest logistic regression model using only a single x-variable can be presented in a table of paired proportional data like the one used for the McNemar test in chapter 3.

	high.....	low leucyte count
Rejections	p_1	$1-p_1$
No rejection	p_2	$1-p_2$

The equation in its simplest version is:

$\ln y = bx$
$b = \ln (p_1(1-p_1)) / \ln (p_2(1-p_2))$
$x = \ln (p_2(1-p_2))$

or

$\ln (p_1(1-p_1)) = \ln (p_1(1-p_1)) / \ln (p_2(1-p_2)) \cdot \ln (p_2(1-p_2))$

$p(1-p)$ = the odds of finding yes-data as explained in the above paired table. The b-value in the logistic regression equation can be best understood as the odds ratio of finding p_1 $(1-p_1)$ given $p_2(1-p_2)$. Although with multiple-variables logistic regression becomes a formidable technique, it is straightforward to understand, and logistic regression increasingly finds its way into the secondary analysis of trial data.

4. CONCLUSIONS

Sometimes it is decided already at the design stage of a clinical trial to perform post-hoc analyses in order to test secondary hypotheses. For the purpose of power we may make two new groups: those who have improvement and those who have not, irrespective of the type of treatment. We, then, can perform a regression analyis of the two new groups trying to find independent determinants of improvement. If one or more determinants for adjustment are binary, which is generally so, our choice of test is logistic regression analysis. This procedure does of course provide no proof. However, it may give strong support for the presence of particular underlying mechanisms in the data.

5. REFERENCES

1. Cleophas TJ, Remmert HP, Kauw FH. Celiprolol versus propranolol in unstable angina pectoris. Clin Pharmacol Ther 1996; 45: 476-73.
2. Van der Vring AF, Cleophas TJ, Zwinderman AH, et al. Different classes of calcium channel blockers in addition beta-blockers for exercise induced angina pectoris. Br J Clin Pharmacol 1999; 50: 545-60.

CHAPTER 15

QUALITY-OF-LIFE ASSESSMENTS IN CLINICAL TRIALS

1.SUMMARY

Background: Two major issues in quality of life (QOL) research include the patients'opinion as a contributing factor in QOL-assessments, and the lack of sensitivity of QOL-assessments.

Objectives: To review results from recent research by the Dutch Mononitrate Quality Of Life (DUMQOL) Study Group relevant to these issues.

Results: Using a test-battery including Stewart's Short Form (SF)-36 Questionnaire and the DUMQOL-50 questionnaire, the DUMQOL Study Group tested the hypothesis that the patients'opinion might be an independent determinant of QOL and performed for that purpose a stepwise multiple regression analysis of data from 82 outpatient clinic patients with stable angina pectoris. Psychological distress was the most important contributor to QOL (beta 0.43, P<0.0001). Also, the patients'opinion significantly contributed to QOL (beta 0.22, P= 0.032). Physical health status according to the patients'judgment only made a borderline contribution (beta 0.19, P=0.71), while the physicians'judgment was not associated with QOL at all (beta 0.11, P=0.87). Using an Odds ratio approach of QOL scores in 1350 outpatient clinic patients with stable angina pectoris the DUMQOL Study Group assessed the question that relative scores might provide increased precision to estimate the effects of patient characteristics on QOL data. Increased QOL difficulties were observed in New York Heart Association Angina Class (NYHA) III-IV patients, in patients with comorbidity, as well as in females and elderly patients. Odds ratios can be used in these categories to predict the benefit from treatments.

Conclusions: Recent QOL-research of the DUMQOL Study Group allows for conclusions relevant to clinical practice. QOL should be defined in a subjective rather than objective way. The patients'opinion is an important independent contributor to QOL. The comparison of absolute QOL-scores lacks sensitivity to truly estimate QOL. The odds ratio approach of QOL scores provides increased precision to estimate QOL.

2. INTRODUCTION

Less than 10 years ago the scientific community believed that quality of life (QOL) was part of the art of medicine rather than the science of medicine. In the past few years index methods have been developed and have proven to be sensitive and specific to assess patients'health status not only on a physical, but also on a psychological and social base. We increasingly witness that QOL is implemented in the scientific evaluation of medicine. However, major problems with QOL assessments so far, include the contributing factor patients'opinion, which is very subjective and, therefore, scientifically difficult to handle, and ,second, the low sensitivity of QOL-questionnaires to reflect true changes in QOL. The Dutch Mononitrate Quality Of Life (DUMQOL) Study Group has recently addressed both problems. In their hands, the patients' opinion was a consistent and statistically independent determinant of QOL in patients with angina pectoris. The problem of low sensitivity of QOL-assessments could be improved by replacing the absolute score-scales with relative ones, using for that purpose odds ratios of scores. The current chapter reviews the main results of this so far only partly published research[1,2] from the Netherlands.

3. SOME TERMINOLOGY

QOL battery

A questionnaire large enough to adequately address important domains of QOL.

Domains of QOL

Physical, psychological , and social areas of health seen as distinct and important to a person's perception of QOL.

Items

Items, otherwise called questions, constitute a domain, e.g., the DUMQOL-questionnaire for angina pectoris, consists of respectively 8, 7, and 4 questions to assess the domains (1) mobility, (2) somatic symptoms, and (3) psychological distress.

Absolute score scales

For every item the individual response is scored on a (linear) scale. Mean of scores a group of patients are calculated. Mean domain scores are calculated as overall means of the latter mean scores.

Relative score scales

The same procedure. However, results are reported in the form of odds ratios.

Odds ratios

Mean of the domain scores in patients with a particular characteristic / mean of the domain scores in patients without this particular characteristic.

Validated QOL batteries	This is controversial. QOL batteries are diagnostic tests, and validation of any diagnostic test is hard to accomplish without a golden standard for comparison. Surrogate validation is sometimes used: actual QOL scores are compared with scores expected based on levels of morbidity.
Internal consistency of domain items	There should be a strong correlation between the answers given to questions within one domain: all of questions should approximately predict one and the same thing. The level of correlation is expressed as Cronbach's alpha: 0 means poor, 1 perfect relationship.
Cronbach's alpha	$alpha = k / (k-1) . (1- \Sigma(s^2_i) / s^2_T)$ $k=$ number of items $s^2_i =$ variance of ith item $s^2_T =$ variance of total score obtained by summing up all of the items
Multicollinearity	There should not be a too strong correlation between different domain scores because different domains predict different areas of QOL. A Pearson's correlation coefficient > 0.90 means the presence of multicollinearity and, thus, of a flawed multiple regression analysis.
Pearson's correlation coefficient (r)	$$r = \frac{\Sigma(x-\bar{x})(y-\bar{y})}{\sqrt{\Sigma(x-\bar{x})^2 (y-\bar{y})^2}}$$
Sensitivity of QOL assessment	Sensitivity or precision means ability of the measurement to reflect true changes in QOL.
QOL estimator	Mean (or pooled) result of the data from a single domain.
Index methods	Index methods combine the results of various domains of a QOL battery to provide an index for overall QOL.

4. DEFINING QOL IN A SUBJECTIVE OR OBJECTIVE WAY?

In 1992 Brazier et al[3] validated the Short Form (SF)-36 health survey questionnaire of Stewart[4] , a self-administered questionnaire, addressing any aspects that, according to the designer, might be important to the patients'QOL. However, at each item in the questionnaire, the question "is it important to you?" was missing. In 1994 Gill and Feinstein[5] in their "Critical appraisal of quality of life assessments" emphasized that, from their personal experience in patient care, they believed that QOL, rather than a description of health status, should describe the way patients perceive their health status. One year later Marquis et al[6] designed a questionnaire for patients with angina pectoris based on psychological factors, in addition to clinical symptoms, and concluded that the former is probably a better predictor of QOL than the latter. In subsequent years QOL assessments increasingly allowed for patients giving their own opinion, in addition to patients answering questions about health status. However, the latter was consistently given more weight than the former. For example, Testa and Simonson[7] allowed for one such question out of 6 questions in each QOL-domain giving the question just about 1/6 of the total weight in various domains. The problem with the subjective approach to QOL, as recently pointed out by Thompson et al[8], is that it is difficult to match with the accepted rule that scientific data should be objective. In addition, the patients'opinion may be a variable so unpredictable, that it cannot be applied as a reliable measure for clinical assessment of groups of patients. So far, the concept that the patients'opinion is a relevant variable in the assessment of QOL has never been proven to be true. In order to test this issue the DUMQOL Study Group has recently completed some relevant research.

5. THE PATIENTS'OPINION IS AN IMPORTANT INDEPENDENT-CONTRIBUTOR TO QOL

The DUMQOL Study Group used the validated form of Stewart's SF-36 Questionnaire for the purpose of scoring QOL[3] , and the DUMQOL-50 questionnaire for scoring psychological distress and health status according to the patients'judgment.[9] The patients' opinion (patients were requested to estimate the overall amount of his/her QOL as compared to patients they knew with a similar condition) and health status according to the physicians'judgement (the physician was requested to estimate the patients'health status) were scored like the others on 5 point-scales. Internal consistency and retreatment reliability of the test-battery was adequate with Cronbach's alpha 0.66. Table 1 shows the results from a cohort of 82 outpatient-clinic

Table 1. Correlation matrix to assess multicollinearity
in the data, Pearson's correlation coefficient are given (r).

	patients' opinion	psychological distress	health status	health status patients' judgment
physicians'judgment				
Psychological distress	0.35			
Health status patients'judgment	0.36	0.30		
Health status physicians'judgment	0.42	0.41	0.48	
Quality of life	0.42	0.58	0.43	0.27

r<0.20 weak correlation; 0.20<r<0.40 moderate correlation; r>0.40 strong correlation

Table 2. Stepwise multiple regression analysis of the associations of various (dependent)
predictors on QOL in patients with angina pectoris

	Beta	T	P- value
Psychological distress	0.43	4.22	0.000
Patients'opinion	0.22	2.19	0.032
Health status (patients'judgment)	0.19	1.88	0.071
Health status (physicians'judgment)	0.11	0.16	0.872

beta= standardized partial correlation coefficient

patients with stable angina pectoris. Obviously, QOL was strongly associated with the patients'opinion. In none of the comparisons were adjustment for multicollinearity required (Pearson's correlation coefficient >0.9). Table 2 shows that psychological distress was the most important contributor to QOL. Also, the patients'opinion significantly contributed to QOL. Physical health status according to the patients'judgment only made a borderline contribution, while the physicians'judgment was not associated with QOL at all. These data strongly support the relevance of the patients'opinion as a important independent-contributor to QOL.

6. LACK OF SENSITIVITY OF QOL-ASSESSMENTS

Sensitivity defined as ability of the measurement to reflect true changes in QOL is frequently poor in QOL assessments.[10] A well-established problem with QOL scales is their inconsistent relationship between ranges of response and true changes in QOL.[7] A good example of this problem is the physical scale of the SF-36 questionnaire. It ranges from 0 to 100 points. However, while healthy youngsters may score as high as 95 and topsporters even 100, 60 year-old subjects usually score no better than 20. A patients with angina pectoris may score 5 points. If he would score 10, instead of 5, after the allowance of sublingual nitrates ad libitum, this improvement would equal 5% on the absolute scale of 100 points, which does not seem to be very much. However, on a relative scale this score of 10 points is 100% better than a score of 5 points, and, in terms of improvement of QOL, this difference on the SF-36-scale between 5 and 10 points does mean a world of difference. It, for example, means the difference between a largely dependent and independent way of life. In this example the low score on the absolute-scale masks important and meaningful changes in QOL. The DUMQOL Study Group took issue with this well-recognized but unsolved phenomenon and performed an odds ratio analysis of patient characteristics in a cohort of 1350 patients with stable angina pectoris. They showed that this approach provided increased precision to estimate effects on QOL estimators.

7. ODDS RATIO ANALYSIS OF EFFECTS OF PATIENT CHARACTERISTICS ON QOL DATA PROVIDES INCREASED PRECISION

Table 3 gives an overview of effects of patient characteristics on QOL estimators in 1350 patients with stable angina pectoris. Results are presented as odds ratios. The odds ratio presents the relative risk of QOL difficulties and is defined as the ratio between mean domain score of patients with a particular characteristic and that of patients without this particular characteristic.

Table 3. Stable angina pectoris: effects of patient characteristics on quality of life estimators. Odds ratios and 95% confidence intervals are given.

	Mobility difficulties	Pain in general	Early morning pain	Psychological distress	Chest pain	Patient satisfaction
Gender (females/males)	2.5 (1.8-3.3)^c	2.0 (1.3-3.0)^c	1.7 (0.6-4.7)	1.3 (0.9-2.0)	2.1 (1.1-3.9)^b	0.8 (0.3-1.9)
Age (>68/<86 years)	1.4 (1.2-1.5)^b	1.0(0.9-1.1)	0.9 (0.9-1.0)	1.0 (0.9-1.0)	1.0 (0.9-1.0)	1.0 (0.9-1.0)
NYHA (III-and-IV / II-and-I)	5.6 (4.8-6.6)^c	2.8 (2.1-3.5)^c	46.8 (26.3-83.1)^c	4.4 (3.5-5.5)^c	37.2 (23.4-58.9)^c	0.6 (0.4-1.1)
Smoking yes/no	0.8 (0.5-1.1)	1.3 (0.8-2.1)	12.9 (3.0-56.2)^c	3.2 (2.0-5.2)^a	0.5 (0.2-1.2)	5.8(2.1-15.8)^b
Cholesterol yes/no	0.9 (0.7-1.3)	1.4 (0.3-2.0)	1.3 (0.5-3.4)	1.8 (1.2-2.8)^a	1.8 (0.9-3.4)	1.1 (0.5-2.6)
Hypertension yes/no	0.3 (0.2-0.4)^a	0.5 (0.3-0.7)^a	0.7 (0.2-0.9)^a	0.3 (0.2-0.4)^b	0.5 (0.3-0.9)^a	1.7 (0.7-4.1)
Diabetes yes/no	2.2 (1.5-3.1)^a	1.1 (0.6-1.9)	9.1 (3.0-28.2)^c	2.0 (1.1-3.7)^a	1.8 (0.7-4.6)	1.1 (0.3-4.2)
Arrhythmias yes/no	2.9 (2.0-4.1)^b	1.3 (0.7-2.1)	3.6 (1.3-10)^a	3.2 (1.9-5.4)^a	10.2 (4.5-23.4)^b	1.2 (0.4-3.7)
PVD yes/no	11.0 (7.9-15.1)^c	2.2 (1.4-3.6)^a	1.1 (0.7-1.7)	2.6 (1.5-4.5)^a	1.0 (0.4-2.2)	8.3 (2.7-25.7)^b
Beta-blockers yes/no	0.8 (0.7-0.9)^a	0.8 (0.5-1.1)	1.7 (0.7-4.0)	0.9 (0.6-1.2)	1.3 (0.7-2.2)	3.2 (1.5-6.9)^b
Calcium channel blockers yes/no	1.5 (1.2-1.9)^a	1.3 (0.9-1.8)	3.2 (1.5-6.6)^a	2.0 (1.4-2.9)^a	6.0 (3.4-10.7)^b	6.5 (3.0-13.8)^a
Sublingual nitrates yes/no	2.6 (2.1-3.3)^c	3.0 (2.2-4.2)^c	1.0 (0.7-1.4)	3.1 (2.5-4.3)^c	7.1 (4.2-12.0)^c	3.4 (1.6-6.9)^c

Quality of life domains were estimated a questionnaire based on the Medical Outcomes Short-Form 36 Health Survey and the Angina Pectoris Quality of Life Questionnaire. Results are given as odds ratios = mean domain scores in patients with characteristic /mean domain scores in patients without characteristic. PVD = peripheral vascular disease; NYHA= New York Heart Association Angina Class; a= P<0.05; b= P<0.01; c= P<0.001.

The procedure readily identifies categories of patients that, obviously, have poor QOL scores. E.g.,

1. Increased QOL-difficulties were observed in patients with advanced New York Heart Association (NYHA) anginal class: the higher the anginal class the larger the risk of mobility difficulties, pain, chest pain, anginal pain, and distress.
2. The risk of mobility difficulties was increased in patients with diabetes mellitus, arrhythmias, and peripheral vascular diseases.
3. Patients using sublingual nitrates (and thus presumably very symptomatic) reported more (severe) mobility difficulties, pain, chest pain, and psychological distress.
4. Female patients reported more (severe) mobility difficulties, pain, anginal pain, and distress than their male counterparts.
5. The risk of mobility difficulties increased with age, but, in contrast, elderly patients reported less pain, anginal pain, and distress.

The above categories of patients are, obviously, very symptomatic and should, therefore, particularly benefit from treatments. The beneficial effects of treatments in patients with particular characteristics can be predicted according to the following procedure:

(1) Odds Ratio $_{active\ treatment\ /\ placebo}$ = mean domain score in patients on active treatment/ mean domain score in patients on placebo.

(2) Odds Ratio $_{characteristic\ /\ no\ characteristic}$ = mean domain score in patients with particular characteristic / mean domain score in patients without this particular characteristic.

The relative risk of scoring in patients with a particular characteristic if they used active treatment

can be estimated and calculated according to:

(3) Odds Ratio $_{characteristic\ /\ no\ characteristic}$ x Odds Ratio $_{active\ treatment\ /\ placebo}$.

Along this line the odds ratio approach to QOL-assessments can be helpful to estimate the effects of cardiovascular drugs on quality of life in different categories of patients with increased precision.

8. DISCUSSION

The medical community is, obviously, attracted to the concept that QOL assessments should pay particular attention to the individual, but, at the same time, it believes in the usefulness of a scientific method to measure QOL.[11] Usually, the objective of a study is not to find the greatest good for a single person but the greatest good for the entire population, moving from an individual perspective to a societal one. Even for quality-of-life measurements, only large clinical studies designed and conducted with rigorous statistical standards allow a hypothesis to be tested and to offer useful results. Using the patients'opinion as measurement-instrument raises a major problem within this context. The general concept of medical measurements is that measurement-instruments remain constant irrespective of who is using them: a thermometer remains the same whoever's mouth it is placed in. With the patients'opinion this is not so. Rather than true ability, perceived functional ability and willingness to complain is assessed. An assessment tool to reflect the viewpoint of patients is, obviously, a major challenge. Although the medical community expresses sympathy with the latter concept, it expresses doubt about scientific value and even questions whether the patients'opinion is part of medicine at all.[7,8,11] The recent research from the DUMQOL Group shows for that the patients'opinion in a standardized way, produces data that are sufficiently homogeneous to enable a sensitive statistical analysis. These data strongly support the relevance of the patients'opinion as a independent contributing factor to QOL. This variable should, therefore, be adequately implemented in future QOL assessments.

A second problem with current QOL-batteries is the inconsistent relationship between ranges of response and true changes in QOL-assessments. This is mainly due to very low (and very high) scores on the absolute-scale, masking important and meaningful changes in QOL. The DUMQOL Study Group showed that this problem can be adequately met by the use of relative rather than absolute scores and used for that purpose an odds ratio-approach of QOL scores. This approach provided increased precision to estimate effects on QOL estimators. An additional advantage of the latter approach is that odds ratios are well understood and much in use in the medical community, and that results from QOL research can, therefore, be more easily communicated through odds ratios than through the comparison of absolute scores. For example, "the odds ratio of (severe) mobility difficulties for mononitrate therapy in patients with stable angina is 0.83 (p<0.001)" is better understood than "the mean mobility difficulties score decreased from 1.10 to 1.06 on a scale from 0 to 4 (p=0.007)".

We conclude that recent QOL-research from the DUMQOL Study Group allows for some relevant conclusions, pertinent to both clinical practice and clinical research. QOL should be assessed in a subjective rather than objective way, because the patients'opinion is an important independent contributor to QOL. The comparison of absolute QOL-scores lacks sensitivity to truly estimate QOL. For that purpose the odds ratio approach of QOL scores provides increased precision to estimate QOL.

9. REFERENCES

1. Frieswijk N, Buunk BP, Janssen RM, Niemeyer MG, Cleophas TJ, Zwinderman AH. Social comparison and quality of life: evaluation in patients with angina pectoris. Cardiogram 2000; 16: 26-31.
2. Zwinderman AH, Niemeyer MG, Kleinjans HA, Cleophas TJ. Application of item response modeling for quality of life assessments in patients with stable angina pectoris. In: Clinical Pharmacology, EDS Kuhlman J, Mrozikiewicz A, Zuckschwerd Verlag, New York, 1999, pp 48 -56.
3. Stewart AL, Hays RD, Ware JE. The MOS short form general health survey. Med Care 1988; 26: 724-735.
4. Brazier JE, Harper R, Jones NM, O'Cathain A, Thomas KJ, Usherwood T, Westlake L, Validating the SF-36 health survey questionnaire: new outcome measure for primary care. Br Med J 1992; 305: 160-164.
5. Gill TM, Feinstein AR. A critical appraisal of the quality of quality-of-life measurements. J Am Med Assoc 1994; 272: 619-626.
6. Marquis P, Fagol C, Joire JE. Quality of life assessment in patients with angina pectoris. Eur Heart J 1995; 16: 1554-1559.
7. Testa MA, Simonson DC. Assessment of quality-of-life outcomes. N Engl J Med 1996; 334: 835 -840.
8. Thompson DR, Meadows KA, Lewin RJ. Measuring quality of life in patients with coronary heart disease. Eur Heart J 1998; 19: 693-695.
9. Niemeyer MG, Kleinjans HA, De Ree R, Zwinderman AH, Cleophas TJ, Van der Wall EE. Comparison of multiple dose and once-daily nitrate therapy in 1350 patients with stable angina pectoris. Angiology 1997; 48: 855-863.
10. Ware JE, Snow KK, Kosinski M, Gandek B. SF-36 Health survey: manual and interpretation guide. Boston. The Health Institute, New England Medical Center, 1993.
11. Albert SM, Frank L, Mrri R, Hylandt, Apolone G, Leplége A. Defining and measuring quality of life in medicine. J Am Med Assoc 1998; 279: 429-431.

CHAPTER 16

STATISTICAL ANALYSIS OF GENETIC DATA

1.INTRODUCTION

In 1860, the benchmark experiments of the monk Gregor Mendel led him to propose the existence of genes. The results of Mendel's pea data were astoundingly close to those predicted by his theory. When we recently looked into Mendel's pea data and performed a chi-square test, we had to conclude the the chi-square value was too small not to reject the null-hypothesis. this would mean that Mendel's reported data were so close to what he expected that we could only conclude that he had somewhat fudged the data.

Table 1. Chi-square-distribution not only has a right but also a left tail. We reject the null - hypothesis of no difference with 1 degree of freedom if chi-square is larger than 3.84 or smaller than 0.004. In Mendel's data frequently very small chi-squares can be observed, as e.g., in the underneath example where it is as small as 0.0039. This means that the chi-square is too small not to reject the null-hypothesis. The results are closer to what can be expected than compatible with the assumption of a normal distribution. The obvious explanation is that Mendel somewhat mispresented his data

Phenotype	A	a
B	AB 27	aB 271
b	Ab 9	ab 93

Though Mendel may have somewhat fudged some of his data, he started a novel science that now 140 years later is the largest growing field in biomedicine. This novel science, although in its first steps, already has a major impact on the lifes of all of us. E.g., obtaining enough drugs, like insulin and many others, to treat illnesses worldwide was a problem that has been solved by recombinant DNA technology which enabled through genetic engineering of bacteria or yeasts the large scale production of various pharmaceutical compounds. The science of genes, often called genomics, is vast, and this chapter only briefly mentions a few statistical techniques developed for processing data of genetic research. We will start with the explanation of a few terms typically used in genomics.

Table 2. Bayes' Theorem, an important approach
for the analysis of genetic data: example

Based on historical data the chance for girls in a particular family of
being carrier for the hemophilia A gene is 50%. Those who are carrier
will have a chance of $1/2 \times 1/2 = \frac{1}{4} = 25\%$ that two sons are healthy. Those
who are no carrier will have a 100 % chance of two healthy sons. This
would mean that a girl from this population who had two healthy sons is
500/125=4 times more likely to be no carrier than to be carrier. In terms
of Bayes'Theorem:
posterior odds = prior odds x likelihood ratio.
prior probability of being carrier= 50%
prior odds= 50:50=1.0
likelihood ratio= probability for carrier of having two healthy sons/
probability for non-carrier of having two healthy sons= 25%/100%=
0.25 posterior odds= 1.0 times 0.25= 25% or 1 in 4:
if you saw many girls from this family you would see one carrier for
every 4 non-carriers.

---

	carrier	no carrier
two sons healthy	n= 125	n=500
two sons not healthy	n=375	n=0

2.SOME TERMINOLOGY

Bayes' Theorem (table 2)	Posterior odds= likelihood ratio x prior odds This approach is required for making predictions from genetic data. Although the general concept of including prior evidence in the statistical analysis of clinical trial data is appealing, this concept should not be applied in usual null-hypothesis testing, because we would have to violate the main assumption of null-hypothesis testing that H0 and H1 have the same frequency distribution.
Posterior odds (table 2)	Prior odds adjusted for likelihood ratio.
Prior odds (table 2)	Prior probability of being a carrier / prior probability of being no carrier.
Likelihood ratio (table 2)	Probability for carriers of having healthy offspring/ probability for non-carrier of having healthy offspring.
Genetic linkage	When 2 genes or DNA sequences are located near each other on the same chromosome, they are linked. When they are not close, crossing over occurs frequently. However, when they are close they tend to be inherited together. Genetic linkage is

useful in genetic diagnosis and mapping because once you know that the disease gene is linked to a particular DNA sequence that is close, the latter can be used as a marker to identify the disease gene indirectly. Bayes' Theorem can be used to combine experimental data with prior linkage probabilities as established.

Autosomal	Not x- or y-chromosome linked.
Heterosomal	X-or y-chromosome linked.
Dominant gene	Gene that is expressed in the phenotype.
Recessive gene	Gene that is expressed in the phenotype only if it is present in two complementary chromosomes.
Haplotype	Group of genetic markers linked together on a single chromosome, such as a group of DNA -sequences.
Haploid genome	Chromosomes of haploid cell (23 chromosomes, 50,000- 100,000 genes).
Diploid cell	Cell with 46 chromosomes.
Chromosome	2,000-5,000 genes.
Chromosomal microband	50-100 genes.
Gene	$1,5-2000.10^3$ base-pairs.
Genomic medicine	Use of genotypic analysis to enhance quality of care.
Complex disease traits	Multifactorial diseases where multiple genes and non-genetic factors interact.
Allele	Gene derived from one parent.
Homozygous	Having identical alleles.
Heterozygous	Having different alleles.
DNA- cloning	Isolation of DNA fragments and their insertion into the nucleic acid from another biologic vector for manipulation.
DNA probe	Cloned DNA fragment used for diagnostic or therapeutic purpose.
Hybridization of single stranded DNA	Double-stranded DNA is dissociated into single -stranded, which can then be used to detect complementary strands.
Blotting procedures	Southern, Northern, Immuno-, Western blotting are all procedures to hybridize target DNA in solution to known DNA-sequences fixed on a membrane support.
Polymerase chain reaction	Oligonucleotide of known nucleic acid sequence is incubated with the target DNA and then amplified with DNA polymerase.
DNA chips	Arrays of oligonucleotides on miniature supports developed for the analysis of unknown DNA sequences, taking advantage of the complementary

	nature of nucleic acid interaction.
Mutations	Changes in DNA either heritable or obtained.
Introns	Non-coding regions of the gene.
Exons	Coding regions of the gene.
Single gene disorders	One gene plays a predominant role in determining disease.
Genotype	Chemical structure of a gene.
Phenotype	Clinical characteristics of a gene.
Gene expression	Regulation of gene function is mediated at a transcriptional level through helix-turn-helix proteins and at a posttranscriptional level through various hormones, autacoids and many more factors.

3. GENETICS, GENOMICS, PROTEONOMICS, DATA MINING

In the past two or three decades the role of genetic determinants have increased enormously in biomedical research. Of several monogenetic diseases the genetic foundation has been clarified almost completely (e.g. Huntington's disease), and of others the contribution of many genetic markers has been proved: for instance the brca 1 and 2 genes in breast cancer[1], and the mismatch gene mutations in coloncarcinoma[2]. Simultaneously, the human genome project has been the catalyst for the development of several high-throughput technologies that have made it possible to map and sequence complex genomes. These technologies are used, and will be used increasingly in clinical trials for many purposes but predominantly to identify genetic variants, and differentially expressed genes that are associated with better or worse clinical efficacy in clinical trials. In addition, the proteins associated with these genes are being investigated to disentangle their roles in the biochemical and physiological pathways of the disease and the treatment that is being studied. Together these technologies are called (high-throughput) genetics, genomics, and proteomics.

The technological advancements have made it possible to measure thousands of genes/proteins of a single patient simultaneously, and the possibility to evaluate the role of each gene/protein in differentiating between e.g. responders and non-responders to therapy. This has increased the statistical problem of multiple testing hugely, but also has stimulated research into statistical methods to deal with it. In addition methods have been developed to consider the role of clusters of genes. In this chapter we will describe a number of these new techniques for the analysis of high throughput genetic data, and for the analysis of gene-expression data. We restrict the discussion to data that are typically sampled in clinical trials including unrelated individuals only. Familial data are extremely important to investigate genetic associations: their clustered structure requires dedicated statistical techniques but these fall outside the scope of this chapter.

4. GENOMICS

In the mid-1970s, molecular biologists developed molecular cloning and DNA sequencing. Automated DNA sequencing and the invention of the polymerase chain reaction (PCR) made it possible to sequence the entire human genome. This has lead to the development of microarrays, sometimes known as DNA-chip technology. Microarrays are ordered sets of DNA molecules of known sequence. Usually rectangular, they can consist of a few hundred to thousands of sets. Each individual feature goes on the array at a precisely defined location on the substrate, and thereafter, labelled cDNA from a test and a reference RNA sample are pooled and co-hybridized. Labelling can be done in several ways, but is usually done with different fluorescently labelled nucleotides (usually Cy5-dCTP for reference, and Cy3-dCTP for test RNA). After stimulation, the expression of these genes can be measured. This involves quantifying the test and reference signals of each fluorophore for each element on the array, traditionally by confocal laser scanning. The ratio of the test and reference signals is commonly used to indicate whether genes have differential expression. Many resources are available on the web concerning the production of microarrays, and about designing microarray experiments (e.g.: 123genomics.homestead.com). A useful textbook is that of Jordan[3].

An example of a microarray is given in Figure 1. This concerns the differential expression of about 500 genes in tumour tissue of a single patient with gastric tumour.

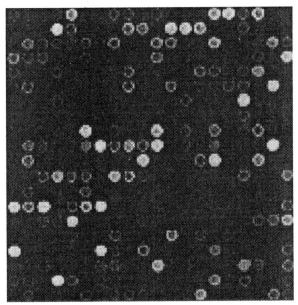

Figure 1. Example of microarray of different expression of about 500 genes in tumour tissue of a single patient.

Each spot in this chip represents a different gene, and the ratio of the two fluorescent dyes indicates whether the genes are over-expressed (red) or under-expressed (green) in the tumour tissue with respect to normal tissue. The transformation of the image into gene expression numbers is not trivial: the spots have to be identified on the chip, their boundaries defined, the fluorescence intensity measured, and compared to the background intensity. Usually this 'image processing' is done automatically by the image analysis software, but sometimes laborious manual adjustments are necessary. One of the most popular systems for image analysis is ScanAlyze (http://rana.stanford.edu/software).

After the image analysis, differential expression is measured by a so-called normalized ratio of the two fluorescence signals, normalized to several experimental factors. The normalized ratios of the array in figure 1 are given in figure 2. On the x-axis are given the 500 genes, and on the y-axis is given the normalized ratio of each gene.

It is obvious that most genes have a ratio around unity, but three or four genes are highly over-expressed with ratios above two. It is typically assumed that ratios

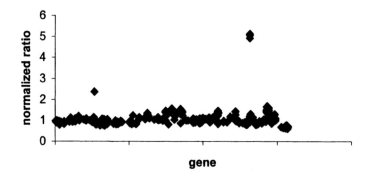

Figure 2. Normalized ratios of the array from figure 1.

larger than 1.5 or 2.0 are indicative of a significant change in gene expression. These estimates are very crude, however, because the reliability of ratios depend on the two absolute intensities. On statistical grounds, moreover, we would expect a number of genes to show differential expression purely by chance[4].
One way of circumventing the multiple testing problem here, is to use a mixture model[5]. Usually, it is assumed that the sample of ratios consists of subgroups of genes with normal, under-, and over-expression. In each subgroup, the ratios are mostly assumed to be normally distributed. When the sample is large enough, the percentage of normal, under-, and over-expressed genes, and associated mean ratios and standard deviations can be estimated from the data. Usually, this is done with the logarithmically transformed ratios. The histogram of the log-transformed ratios

in figure 2 is given in Figure 3, together with the three estimated normal distributions. In this model the probability of each gene of being over- of under-expressed can be calculated using Bayes' theorem.

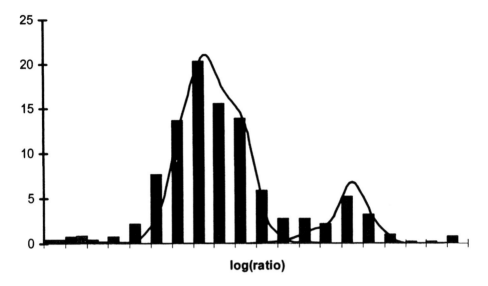

log(ratio)

Figure 3. The histogram of the log-transformed ratios from figure 2, calculated according to bayes 'Theorem.

Although under-expressed genes could not be   identified in this case, over-expressed genes were clearly seen, represented by the second mode to the right. Actually it was estimated that 14% of the genes showed over-expression, corresponding with ratios larger than 1.3.

Above is illustrated how to look at the data of a single microarray. For the analysis of a set of microarrays several different approaches are used. Two distinctions can be used: supervised or unsupervised data analysis, and hypotheses-driven or datamining. For supervised data analysis additional data must be available to which the expression data can be related. In clinical trials a major question is often how responders and non-responders can be distinguished. Relating such response data to expression data can be done using well known techniques such as discriminant-analysis, or logistic regression. Since there may be hundreds or thousands of expression variables, one must be careful in applying these techniques, and cross-validation is often extremely useful[6]. Unsupervised data analysis is usually done by cluster analysis or principal component analysis to find groups of co-regulated genes or related samples. These techniques are often applied without specific prior knowledge on which genes are involved in which case the analysis is a kind of datamining. An example of a hypothesis driven analysis is to pick a potential interesting gene, and then find a group of similar or anti-correlated expression profiles.

Cluster-analysis is the most popular method currently used as the first step in gene expression analysis. Several variants have been developed: hierarchical[7], and k-means[8] clustering, self-organizing maps[9], and gene-shaving[10], and there are many more. All aim at finding groups of genes with similar properties. These techniques can be viewed as a dimensionality reduction technique, since the many thousands of genes are reduced to a few groups of similarly behaving genes. Again many tools are available on the web, and a useful site to start searching is: www.microarray.org. We used Michael Eisen's package[7] to cluster the expression data of 18 patients with gastric cancer. The typical output of a hierarchical clustering analysis is given in Figure 4. This is a dendogram illustrating the similarities between patients, a similar graph can be obtained illustrating similarities between genes. In the present case one might conclude that patients 2,6,5,7,3,13,9,10,1 and 8 form a cluster, and patients 14,15,4,11,16,17,12, and 18 another cluster. But identifying more clusters may be meaningful too.

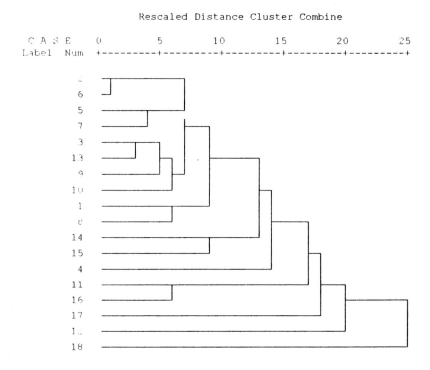

Figure 4. The typical hierarchical clustering analysis of the expression data of 18 patients with gastric cancer.

In a K-means cluster analysis the number of clusters must be specified a priori. When we specify two clusters, the same solution is found as above.

The above results illustrate that many subjective decisions need to be made in a cluster analysis, and such analysis cannot be regarded as hypothesis-driven; the primary output of a cluster analysis are new hypotheses concerning differential expressions.

5. CONCLUSIONS

Although high throughput methods are still relatively expensive, and are not used routinely in clinical trials, these methods undoubtedly will be used more often in the future. Their promise of identifying subgroups of patients with varying drug response is of major importance and is a major topic of pharmaco-genomics. In addition, differential expression profiles, and proteomics are of major importance of identifying new pathways for targeting new drugs. More sophisticated statistical methods are required, and will be developed.

6.REFERENCES

1.Cornelisse CJ, Cornelis RS, Devilee P. Genes responsible for familial breast cancer. Pathol Res Pract 1996 Jul;192(7):684-93.
2.Wijnen JT, Vasen HF, Khan PM, Zwinderman AH, van der Klift H, Mulder A, Tops C, Moller P, Fodde R. Clinical findings with implications for genetic testing in families with clustering of colorectal cancer. N Engl J Med 1998 Aug 20;339(8):511-8 .
3.Jordan B (Ed.). DNA Microarrays: gene expression applications. Berlin: Springer-Verlag, 2001.
4.Claverie JM. Computional methods for the identification of differential and coordinated gene expression. Hum Mol Genet 2001; 8 (10): 1821-32.
5.McLachlan G. Mixture.model clustering of microarray expression data. Aus Biometrics and New Zealand Stat Association Joint Conference, 2001, Christchurch, New Zealand.
6.Alizadeh et al. Distinct types of diffuse large B-cell lymphoma identified by gene expression profiling. Nature 2000, 403: 503-11.
7.Eisen M et al. Cluster analysis and display of genome-wide expression patterns. Proc Natl Acad Sci USA, 1998, 95: 14863-7.
8.Tavazoie et al. Sustematic determination of genetic network architecture. Nat Genet 1999, 22: 281-5.
9.Tamayo et al. Interpreting patterns of gene-expression with self-organizing maps. Proc Natl Acad Sci USA, 1999, 96: 2907-12.

10. Tibshirani et al. Clustering methods for the analysis of DNA microarray data. Tech. rep. Stanford University, Dept of Statistics, Stanford.

CHAPTER 17

RELATIONSHIP AMONG STATISTICAL DISTRIBUTIONS

1.SUMMARY

Background: Statistical analyses of clinical data are increasingly complex. They often involve multiple groups and measures. Such data can not be assessed simply by differences between means but rather by comparing variances.

Objective: To focus on the Chi-square (χ^2)-test as a method to assess variances and test differences between variances. To give examples of clinical data where the emphasis is on variance. To assess interrelation between Chi-square and other statistical methods like normal-test (Z-test), T-test and Analysis-Of-Variance (ANOVA).

Results: A Chi-square-distribution is nothing else than the distribution of square values of a normal-distribution. Null-hypothesis-testing-of-variances is much similar to null-hypothesis-testing-of-means. With the latter we reject the null-hypothesis of no effect if our mean is more than 1.96 SEMs (standard errors of the mean) distant from zero. With the latter we reject the null-hypothesis of no effect if our standardized variance is more than 1.96^2 SEMs² distant from zero. Because variances are squared and, thus, non-negative values, the Chi-square approach can be extended to test hypotheses about many samples. When variances or add-up variances of many samples are larger than allowed for by the Chi-square-distribution-graphs, we reject the probability that our results are from normal distributions, and conclude that our results are significantly different from zero. The Chi-square test is not only adequate to test multiple samples simultaneously, but is also the basis of analysis of variance (ANOVA).

Conclusions: The Chi-square-distribution focused on in this paper is just another approach of the bell-shape-like normal-distribution and is also the basic element of the F-distribution as used in ANOVA. Having some idea about interrelations between these distributions will be of help in understanding benefits and limitations of Chi-square-statistic and its many extensions for the analysis of experimental clinical data.

2.INTRODUCTION

Samples of clinical data are frequently assessed through 3 variables:

The mean result of the data.

The spread or variability of the data.

The sample size.

Generally, we are primarily interested in the first variable, but mean or proportion does not tell the whole story, and the spread of the data may be more relevant. For example, when studying how two drugs reach various organs, the mean level may be the same for both, but one drug may be more variable than the other. In some cases, too little and, in other cases, dangerously high levels get through. The Chi-square-distribution, unlike the normal distribution, is used for the assessment of such variabilities. Clinical scientists although they are generally familiar with the concept of null-hypothesis-testing of normally distributed data, have difficulties to understand the null-hypothesis testing of Chi-square-distributed data, and do not know how closely Chi-square is related to the normal-distribution or the T-distribution. The Chi-square-distribution has a relatively young history. It has been invented by K. Pearson [1] one hundred years ago, three hundred years after the invention of the normal-distribution (A. de Moivre 1667-1754). The Chi-square-distribution and its extensions have become the basis of modern statistics and have provided statisticians with a relatively simple device to analyze complex data, including multiple groups and multivariate analyses. The present paper was written for clinical investigators / scientists in order to better understand the relation between normal and chi-square distribution, and how they are being applied for the purpose of null-hypothesis testing.

3.VARIANCES

Repeated observations exhibit a central tendency, the mean, but, in addition, exhibit spread or dispersion, the tendency to depart from central tendency. If measurement of central tendency is thought of as good bets, then measures of spread represent the poorness of central tendency otherwise called deviation or error. The larger such deviations are, the more do cases differ from each other and the more spread does the distribution show. What we need is an index to reflect this spread or variability. First of all, why not simply take the average of the deviations (d′s) about the mean as measure of variability:

$$\Sigma d \ /n \text{ where } n= \text{sample size.}$$

This, however, will not work, because when we add up negative and positive departures from the mean, our overall variance will equal zero. A device to get around this difficulty is to take the square of each deviation:

$$\Sigma d^2 \ /n \text{ is defined the variance of n observations.}$$

Σd /n, although it can not be used as index to reflex variability, can be readily used to define the mean of a sample of repeated observations, if the size of observations is taken as distance from zero rather than mean. Suddenly, means and variances look a lot the same, and it is no surprise that statistical curves and tables used to assess either of them are closely related. A Chi-square-distribution is nothing else than the distribution of square values of a normal-distribution. It takes a little matrix-algebra, but it is not hard to prove that if Σd /n = 3, then Σd^2 /n = 9. Null-hypothesis-testing-of-variances is much similar to null-hypothesis-testing-of-means. With the latter we reject the null-hypothesis of no effect if our mean is more than

1.96 SEMs (standard errors of the mean) distant from zero. With the latter we reject the null-hypothesis of no effect if our standardized variance is more than 1.96^2 SEMs^2 distant from zero. Because variances are squared and, thus, non-negative values, the Chi-square approach can be extended to test hypotheses about many samples. When variances or add-up variances of many samples are larger than allowed for by the Chi-square-distribution-graphs, we reject the probability that our results are from normal distributions, and conclude that our results are significantly different from zero. The Chi-square test is not only adequate to test multiple samples simultaneously, but is also the basis of analysis of variance (ANOVA).

4.THE NORMAL DISTRIBUTION

The normal distribution curve can be drawn from the formula below.

$F(x) = 1/\sqrt{2\pi s^2} / e^{-(x-m)/2s}$ where s = standard deviation and m = mean value.

Repeated observations in nature do not precisely follow this single mathematical formula, and may even follow largely different patterns. The formula is just an approximation. And so, it is remarkable that the approach works in practice, although the p-values obtained from it are sometimes given inappropriate emphasis. We should not forget that a p-value of <0.001 does not mean that we have proven something for the entire population, but rather that we have proven something on the understanding that our data follow a normal distribution and that our data are representative for the entire population. Frequently, the results as provided by clinical trials are much better than those observed in general practice, because the population follows a different frequency distribution or because the enrollees in a trial are selected groups not representative for the entire population. We wish that more often these possibilities would be accounted by the advocates of evidence-based medicine. If we are willing to accept the above limitations, the normal distribution can be used to try and make predictions, with the understanding that statistical testing cannot give certainties, only chances. How was the normal distribution invented? At first, investigators described their data in the form of histograms (Figure 1 upper graph: on the x-axis the individual data and on the y-axis how often).

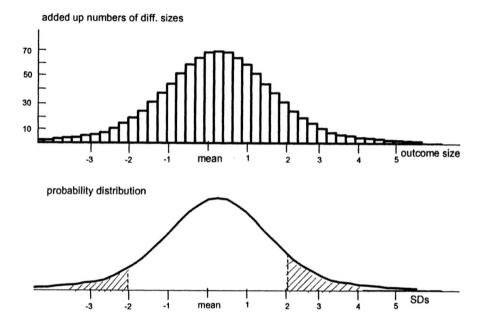

Figure 1. *Upper graph shows histogram: on the x-axis we have the individual data and on the y-axis we have "how often" (the mean value is observed most frequently, while the bars on both side of the mean gradually grew shorter). Lower graph shows normal distribution: the bars on the y-axis have been replaced by a continuous line, it is now impossible to read from the graph how many patients had a particular outcome. Instead, we infer that the total area under the curve (AUC) represents 100% of our data, AUC left from the mean represents 50%, left from -1SD (standard deviation) 15% of the data, and left from -2 SDs 2.5 % of the data. This curve although suitable for describing a sampe of repeated observations, is not yet adequate for testing statistical hypotheses.*

Often, the mean value was observed most frequently, while the bars on both side of the mean gradually grew shorter. From this histogram to a normal distribution curve is a short step (Figure 1 lower graph). The bars on the y-axis have been replaced by a continuous line. It is now impossible to read from the graph how many patients had a particular outcome. Instead, relevant inferences can be made: the total area under the curve (AUC) presents 100% of our data, AUC left from the mean presents 50%, left from - 1SD (standard deviation) 15% of the data, and left from -2 SDs 2.5 % of the data. This curve although suitable for describing a sampe of repeated observations, is not yet adequate for testing statistical hypotheses. For that purpose, a narrow normal curve is required (Figure 2).

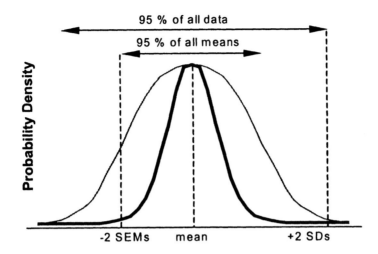

Figure 2. Narrow and wide normal curve: the wide one summarizes the data of our trial, the narrow one summarizes the means of many trials similar to our trial.

The narrow and wide curve from Figure 2 are both based on the same data, but have different meaning. The wide (with SDs on the x-axis) one summarizes the data of our trial, the narrow one (with SEMs (standard errors of the mean) on the x-axis) summarizes the means of many trials similar to ours. This may be difficult to understand, but it is easy to conceive that the distributions of means of many trials will be narrower and have fewer outliers than the distribution of the actual data. This concept is relevant, because we want to use it for making predictions from our data to the entire population.

We should add here that there is only a small difference between the normal and the T distribution. The latter is a bit wider with small numbers. The chi-square distribution makes no difference between normally and T-like distributed data.

5. NULL-HYPOTHESIS TESTING WITH THE NORMAL OR T-DISTRIBUTION

What does "null-hypothesis" mean: it means that we hypothesize that the result of our trial is not different from zero, we have a negative trial. What does the null-hypothesis look like in graph? Figure 3 shows H1, the graph based on the data of our trial with SEMs on the x-axis (z-axis), and H0, the same graph with a mean of 0.

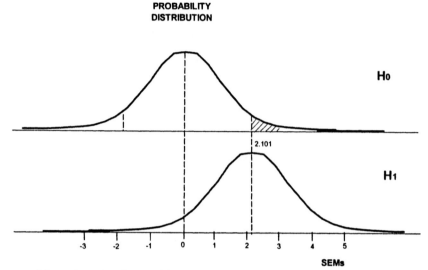

**PROBABILITY
DISTRIBUTION**

***Figure 3.** H1 is the graph based on the data of our trial with SEMs on the x-
axis (z-axis) and H0 is the same graph with mean 0 (mean ± SEM= 0 ± 1).*

Now we make a giant leap from our data to the entire population, and we can do so,
because we assume, that our data are representative for the entire population. H1 is
also the summary of the means of many trials similar to our trial. If we repeated the
trial, differences would be small and the summary would look alike. H0 is also the
summary of the means of many trials similar to our trial, but with an overall effect
of 0. Our mean is not 0, but 2.9. Still it could be an outlier of may studies with an
overall effect of 0. So, think from now on of H0 as distribution of the means of
many trials with overall effect 0. If hypothesis 0 is true, then the mean of our study
is part of H0. We can not prove this, but we can calculate the chance/probability of
this possibility. A mean result of 2.9 is far distant from 0. Suppose it belongs to H0.
Only 5% of the H0-trials are more than 2.1 SEMs distant from 0, because the AUC
of H0 = 5%. Thus, the chance that it belongs to H0 is less than 5%. We reject the
null-hypothesis of no effect concluding that there is less than 5% chance to find this
result. In usual terms, we reject the null-hypothesis of no effect at p<0.05 or <5%.

6. RELATIONSHIP BETWEEN THE NORMAL-DISTRIBUTION AND CHI-SQUARE-DISTRIBUTION, NULL-HYPOTHESIS TESTING WITH CHI-SQUARE DISTRIBUTION

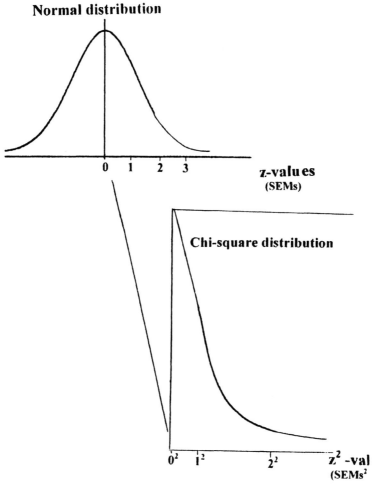

Figure 4. Upper graph shows a normal distribution. Lower graph shows what happens if the x-values of this normal-like-curve are squared The normal-curve changes into a Chi-square-curve.

The upper graph of Figure 4 shows a normal distribution, on the x-axis individual data expressed as distances from the mean, and on the y-axis "how often" the individual data are being observed. The lower graph of Figure 4 shows what happens of the x-values of this normal distribution with mean zero are squared. We get no negative x-values anymore, and the x-values 0 and 1 give rise to y-values twice the size, while the new curve is skewed to the right: the n₋⁻   ·ırve is what we call a chi-square curve. The upper curve is used to test the null-hypothesis that the mean result of our trial is significantly different from zero, the lower one to test that our variance is significantly different from zero.

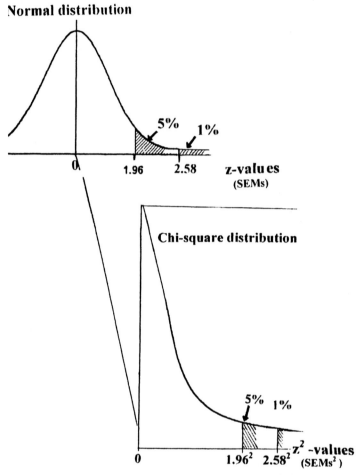

Figure 5. Upper graph gives the x-values, otherwise called Z-values, of a null-hypothesis of a real normal-distribution. Lower graph shows what happens when Z-values are squared. The Z-distribution turns into a non-negative Chi-square- distribution. Upper graph: with $z > 1.96$ $\Delta AUC < 5\%$; lower graph: with $z^2 > (1.96)^2$ $\Delta AUC < 5\%$.

Figure 5 shows how things work in practice. The upper graph gives on the x-axis the possible mean result or our trial expressed in units of SEMs, otherwise called z-value, or, with T-test, T-value. On the y-axis we "how often this result will be obtained". For example, if our mean result is more than 1 SEM distant from zero, this will happen in 31.7% of the cases, because the area under the curve (AUC) distant from 1 SEM = 31.7%. If our mean result is more than approximately 2 SEMs (or with normal distribution precisely 1.96 SEMs) distant from zero, this will happen in 5% of the cases, because the AUC distant from 1.96 SEMs is 5%. If more than 2.58 distant from zero, this will happen in 1% of the cases. With a result that far from zero we reject the null-hypothesis that our result is not different from 0, and conclude that, obviously, our data are significantly different from 0, at p<5% or 1% (<0.05 or <0.01).

Figure 5 lower graph gives a draft of the possible variances of our trial. On the x-axis we have the variance of our trial expressed in units $(SEMs)^2$, otherwise called z^2- values. On the y-axis we have again "how often this variance will be obtained". For example, if our variance is more than 1.96^2 $SEMs^2$ distant from zero, this will happen in less than 5% of the cases. This is so, because the AUC right from $z^2 = 1.96^2$ is 5% of the total AUC of 100%. If our variance is more than $z^2 = 2.58^2$ distant from zero, this chance is 1%. We reject the null-hypothesis that our variance is not significantly different from 0 and we do so at a probability of 1% (p<0.01).

7. EXAMPLES OF DATA WHERE VARIANCE IS MORE IMPORTANT THAN MEAN.

The effects on circadian glucose levels of slow-release-insulin and acute-release-insulin are different. The mean glucose-level is the same for both treatment formulas, but the latter formula produces more low and high glucose levels. Spread or variance of the data is a more important determinant of treatment effect than is the mean glucose value.

A pill producing device is approved only if it will produce pills with a SD not larger than e.g. 6mg. Rather than mean the variance of a test-sample is required to test the device.

Anxious people may not only show a lower average of performance, but also a higher variability in performance relative to their non-anxious counterparts. Variance, in addition to average of performance is required to allow for predictions on performances.

For hospital managers the variability in stay-days in hospital is more relevant than the mean stay-days, because greater variability is accompanied with a more demanding type of care.

A clinician needs to know whether variability in rectal temperature is larger than variability in oral temperature.

Why should we statistically test such questions anyway? Or why not simply calculate the mean result and standard deviation of a sample of data, and, then, check if the SD is within a predefined area. We, subsequently, accept this as sufficient probability to make further predictions about future observations. However, by doing so we will never know the size of this probability. A statistical test rejects the null-hypothesis of no difference from 0 at a 5 % or lower level of probability, and this procedure is widely valued as a powerful aid to erroneous conclusions.

8.CHI-SQUARE CAN BE USED FOR MULTIPLE SAMPLES OF DATA

Unlike the normal-test or the T-test, the Chi-square-test can be extended to testing more than one sample of data simultaneously. Variances are non-negative values, and they can simply be added up. This is, actually, the way variance is defined, the add-up sum of squared distances from the mean. Any subsequent sample of data, if from a normal distribution or T-distribution can be simply added up to the first sample and the add-up sum can be analyzed simultaneously. And, so, with little more effort than demonstrated for 1 sample of data, multiple samples can be added to the model in order to test the null-hypothesis of no difference from zero. This is possible both for samples of continuous data and proportional data, including percentages, proportions, odds ratios, risk ratios etc. The only difference is the breath of the chi-square curve: it gets wider and wider the more samples or the more proportions we add (Figure 6).

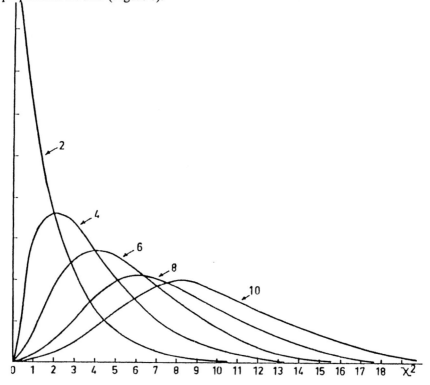

Figure 6.   *The general form of the Chi-square distributions for larger samples of data.*

CONTINGENCY TABLES
The simplest extension of the chi-square test is the analysis of a two-by-two contingency table. With contingency tables we want to test whether two groups of

binary data (yes/no data) are significantly different from one another. We have 4 cells ((1) group-1 yes, (2) group-1 no, (3) group-2 yes, (4) group-2 no). The null-hypothesis is tested by adding up:

chi-square $= (O-E)_{cell\ 1}^2 + (O-E)_{cell\ 2}^2 + (O-E)_{cell\ 3}^2 + (O-E)_{cell\ 4}^2$

where O means observed numbers, and E means expected numbers per cell if no difference between the two groups is true (the null-hypothesis).

HETEROGENEITY BETWEEN RELATIVE RISKS OR ODDS RATIOS IN A META-ANALYSIS OF MULTIPLE TRIALS

In meta-analyses of clinical trials before pooling the results we want to know whether the trials included are heterogeneous or not. A wide add-up variance between trials means that the trials must be from different populations or used different methods and that pooling their results simply is unwarranted. Chi-square-statistic is adequate to assess such questions while natural logarithm is used to approximate normality.

chi-square$= \ln RR_1/s_1^2 + \ln RR_2/s_2^2 + \ln RR_3/s_3^2 + ...$where RR means relative risk and s means SD of this relative risk per sample.

ANALYSIS OF VARIANCE (ANOVA)

A further extension of the use of the Chi-square-statistic is ANOVA. ANOVA makes use of the division-sum of two Chi-square-distributions. This division-sum, indeed, looks much like a usual Chi-square-distribution , as shown for example in Figure 7.

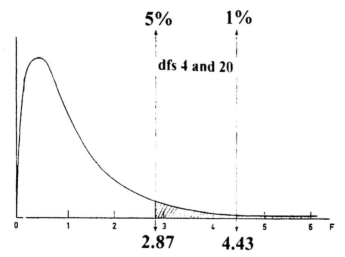

Figure 7. Example of a F-distribution making use of the division-sum of two Chi-square-distributions with 4 and 20 degrees of freedom (dfs).

For example, ANOVA with k groups works as follows:

$$Total\ variation$$
$$|\qquad\qquad|$$

Between-group-variation   within-group-variation

Variations are expressed as sums of squares (SS) and can be added up to obtain the total variation.

We assess whether between-group-variation is large compared to within-group-variation.

Group	n patients	mean	sd
1	-	-	-
2	-	-	-
3	-	-	-
...			
k			

Grand mean = (mean 1 + 2 +3+..k)/k

$$SS_{between\ groups} = n_1\,(\ mean_1 - grand\ mean)^2 + n_2\,(\ mean_2 - grand\ mean)^2 + ...$$
$$SS_{within\ groups} = (n_1-1)(sd_1^{\ 2}\ ) + (n_2-1)\ sd_2^{\ 2} + ...$$

$$F = test\text{-}statistic = \frac{SS_{between\ groups}\ /\ dfs^{xx}}{SS_{within\ groups}\ /\ dfs}$$

[xx]dfs means degrees of freedom (for SS between groups dfs=k-1, for SS within groups dfs=$n_1+n_2+n_3+..n_k-k$).

The F-table gives P-value.

9.CONCLUSIONS

The current chapter is not a cook-book-like instruction for the use of various statistical methods. It only briefly examines the connection between the Chi-square-distribution and other important statistical distributions. They form the basis of all statistical inferences, which are given so much emphasis in today's clinical medicine. The Chi-square-distribution is directly derived from the normal-distribution. The F-distribution is directly derived from the Chi-square distribution. Over and over again, these distributions have shown their utility in the solution of problems in statistical inference. However, none of these distributions is empirical in the sense that someone has taken a large number of samples and found that the sample values actually follow the same mathematical function. Of course, nature does not follow a single mathematical function. The function is an approximation, but it performs well and has proven to be helpful in making clinical predictions. The distribution is also based on assumptions, and, like other theory-based assessments, deals with " if-then" statements. That is why the assumptions about representative samples and normal-distribution in our sample are so important. If we apply the theory of statistics for making inferences from samples, we cannot expect this theory to provide us with adequate answers unless conditions specified in the theory hold true.

Apart from the general requirement of random sampling of independent observations, the most usual assumption made is that the population-distribution is normal. The Chi-square, the T-, and the F-distributions all rest upon this assumption. The normal-distribution can be considered the "parent" distribution to the others. Similarly, there are close connections between the F-distribution and both the normal- and the Chi-square-distributions. Basically, the F-statistic is the ratio of two independent Chi-square-statistics, each of which characterized by its own degrees of freedom. Since a Chi-square-statistic is defined in terms of a normal-distribution, the F-distribution also rests upon the same assumptions, albeit of two (or more than two) normal-distributions. The Chi-square-distribution focused on in this paper is, thus, just another approach of the bell-shape-like normal distribution and and is also the basic element of the F-distribution. Having some idea of the interrelations of these distributions will be of help in understanding how the Chi-square is used to test a hypothesis-of-variance, and how the F-distribution is used to test a hypothesis-about-several-variances.

We conclude that the Chi-square-distribution and its extensions have become the basis of modern statistics and have provided clinical scientists with a relatively simple device to analyze complex data, including multiple groups / multiple variances. The present chapter was written for clinical investigators/ scientists in order to better understand benefits and limitations of Chi-square-statistic and its many extensions for the analysis of experimental clinical data.

10. REFERENCES

1.Pearson K. On a criterion that a given system of deviations from the probable in the case of a correlated system of variables is such that it cannot be reasonably supposed to have arisen from random sampling. Philosophical Magazine 1900; 50: 339-357.

CHAPTER 18

STATISTICS IS NOT "BLOODLESS" ALGEBRA

1. INTRODUCTION

Because biological processes are full of variations, statistics can not give you certainties, but only chances. What kind of chances? Basically, the chances that prior hypotheses are true or untrue. The human brain excels in making hypotheses. We make hypotheses all the time, but they may be untrue. E.g., when you were a kid, you thought that only girls could become doctors, because your family doctor was a girl. Later on this hypothesis appeared to be untrue. In clinical medicine we currently emphasize that hypotheses may be equally untrue and must be assessed prospectively with hard data. That's where statistics comes in, and that's where at the same time many a clinician starts to become nervous, loses his/her self-confidence, and is more than willing to leave his/her data to the statistical consultant who subsequently runs the data through a whole series of statistical tests of SAS[1] or SPSS[2] or comparable statistical computer software to see if there are any significancies. The current article was written to emphasize that the above scenario of analyzing clinical trial data is bad practice and frequently kills the data, and that biostatistics can do more for you than provide you with a host of irrelevant P-values.

2. STATISTICS IS FUN BECAUSE IT PROVES YOUR HYPOTHESIS WAS RIGHT

Statistics is fun, particularly, for the clinical investigator. It is not mathematics, but a discipline at the interface of biology and mathematics. This means that maths is used to answer the biological questions. The scenario as described above does not answer reasonable biological questions. It is called data dredging and is the source of a lot of misinterpretations in clinical medicine. A statistical analysis should be confined to testing of the prior hypotheses. The problem with multiple statistical tests can be explained by gambling 20 times with a chance of success of 5%. You can be sure that after the game you will get $(1-0.05)^{20} = (0.95)^{20} = 0.36 = 36\%$ chance to win a prize. This result is, however, not based on any significant effect but rather on the play of chance. Now, don't let it happen to your trial. Also, a statistical result that does not confirm your prior belief, don't trust it. Make sure that the simplest univariate tests are used for your prospective trial data, because they are adequate and provide the best power. Fancy multivariate procedures are not in place to answer your prior hypotheses. Statistics is fun, because it generally confirms or largely confirms your prior hypotheses, which is appropriate because they were based on sound clinical arguments. If they don't, this is peculiar and should make you anxious to find out why so: imperfections within the design or execution of the trial?[3] It is fun to prove your hypothesis was right, or to find out what you did overlook. Another fun thing with statistics, although completely different and by far not so important, is the method of secondary analyses: it does not prove anything, but it is kind of sports and gives you new and sound ideas for further research.

3. STATISTICAL PRINCIPLES CAN HELP TO IMPROVE THE QUALITY OF THE TRIAL

Over the past decades, the randomized controlled trial has entered an era of continuous improvement and has gradually become accepted as the most effective way of determining the relative efficacy and toxicity of a new therapy because it controls for placebo and time effects. However, even sensitive and properly designed and executed trials do not always confirm hypotheses to be tested, and conclusions are not always confirmed by subsequent trials. Although the former may be due to wrong hypotheses,
the latter is likely to be due to the presence of certain imperfections within the design and execution, and analysis of the trial itself. Such principles could include[4] : (1) giving every effort to avoid asymmetries in the treatment groups [chapter 1, stratification issues], (2) emphasis on statistical power rather than just null-hypothesis testing [chapter 5], (3) assessing asymmetries of outcome variables in order to determine the most important determinants of clinical benefit [chapter 14], (4) accounting routinely for Type III errors of mistakenly believing that an inferior treatment is superior [chapter 5], (5) routinely weighing the odds of benefits against the odds of risks of new treatments.

4. STATISTICS CAN PROVIDE WORTHWHILE EXTRAS TO YOUR RESEARCH

The classical two-parallel-groups design for clinical drug trials is a rather dull activity and is, essentially, unable to answer many current scientific questions. Also, it is laborious, and in the clinical setting sometimes ethically or financially impossible. Examples of what the classical clinical trial design cannot manage: (1) assess multimodal therapies, (2) account historical data, (3) safeguard ethics and efficacy during the course of long-term trials, (4) study drugs, before well-established toxicity information is available, (5) account the possibility of therapeutic equivalence between test and reference treatment, (6) study multiple treatments in one trial, (7) adjust change scores for baseline levels. Alternative designs for such purposes: (1) factorial designs [chapter 1][5], (2) historical controls designs [chapter 1][6], (3) group-sequential interim analysis designs [chapter 6][7], (4) sequential designs for continuous monitoring [chapter 6][8], (5) therapeutic equivalence designs [chapter 4], (6) multiple crossover-periods / multiple parallel-groups designs[9], (7) increased precision designs through multivariate adjustment [chapter 9]. There is, of course, the increased risks of type I/II errors, and the possible loss of some of the validity criteria with the novel designs. However, provided that such possibilities are adequately accounted for in the design stage of the trial, the novel designs are acceptedly valid, and offer relevant scientific, ethical, and financial extras.

5. STATISTICS IS NOT LIKE ALGEBRA BLOODLESS

Statistics is not like algebra bloodless, and requires a lot of biological thinking and just a little bit of mathematics. For example, mathematically we need representative sample sizes to make meaningful inferences about the whole population. Yet, from a biological point of view, this is less true: the first datum encountered in a clinical situation of complete ignorance provides the greatest amount of information from any one datum an investigator will encounter. E.g., consider a new disease for which there is no knowledge whatsoever about the order of magnitude of time of exposure, time of incubation, time of appearance of subsequent symptoms. The first patient for whom we know such data provides a great deal of information.

Another example of biological rather than mathematical thinking involves the issue of making the test parameters alpha and beta flexible. They are mostly set at respectively 5 and 20%. A 20% beta is, however, larger than is appropriate in many cases. E.g., when the false positive is worse for the patient than the false negative, as in case of testing a drug for non-life threatening illness with the drug having severe side effects, the 5 and 20% choices for alpha and beta are reasonable. However, in testing treatment for cancer, the rate of false negatives is worse for the patient, and so, the ratio beta/alpha should be reduced.

A third example of biological thinking is the inclusion of a " safety factor" when estimating prior to a trial the sample size required. Usually the required sample size is calculated from a pilot study or from results quoted in the literature. However, these data are not the actual data from our study, and not using the real data may introduce an error. Also, the data as used for sample size calculation are subject to randomness error. Due to such errors the alpha and beta errors upon which our sample size is based may be larger than we thought. Because of these possibilities we should add a "safety factor" to the sample size as calculated, and make our sample size somewhat larger than the calculated one, e.g., 10 % larger. This is more important, the more uneasy we are about the ultimate result of the study being in agreement with the estimate used for sample size calculation.

6. STATISTICS CAN TURN ART INTO SCIENCE

Traditionally, the science of medicine is considered to be based on experimental evidence, while the art of science is supposed to be based on trust, sympathy, the threatened patient, and other things that no one would believe that could ever be estimated by statistical methods. It is true that factors, of psychosocial and personal nature, are difficult to measure, but it is not impossible to do so. At first, quality of life assessments were based on the amount of primary symptoms, e.g., pain scores etc. Increasingly it is recognized that it should be based on factors like feeling of well-being, social performance. Along this line of development, the art of medicine is more and more turned into science, e.g., with modern quality of life assessments addressing general feeling of well-being, physical activity domains etc. Statistical analyses can be readily performed on validated quality of life indices or any other measurements of effectiveness as developed [chapter 15]. It follows that this development is going to accomplish something that was only shortly believed to be impossible: turning the art of medicine into the science of medicine.

7.STATISTICS FOR SUPPORT RATHER THAN ILLUMINATION?

In 1948 the first randomized controlled trial was published.[10] Until then, observations had been largely uncontrolled. Initially, trials frequently did not confirm hypotheses to be tested. This phenomenon was attributed to little sensitivity due to small samples, as well as inappropriate hypotheses based on biased prior trials. Additional flaws were being recognized and, subsequently better accounted for: carryover effects due to insufficient washout from previous treatments, time effects due to external factors and the natural history of conditions being studied, bias due to asymmetry between treatment groups, lack of sensitivity due to a negative correlation between treatment responses etc. Currently, due to the complexity of trials, clinicians increasingly leave the thinking to statisticians, a practice which is essentially wrong and produces flawed research, because bio-research requires a lot of biological thinking and no more than a bit of statistics. Moreover, a statistician can do much more for you than provide you with a host of irrelevant P-values, but he/she can only do so, if you intuitively know what statistics can and what it cannot answer. Like Prof. M.Hills, the famous statistician of London, used to say, clinicians often use statistics as a drunk uses a lantern standard, for support rather than illumination. Illumination can be obtained by exploring your clinical intuition against a non-mathematical background.

8. STATISTICS CAN HELP THE CLINICIAN TO BETTER UNDERSTAND LIMITATIONS AND BENEFITS OF CURRENT RESEARCH

Medical literature is currently snowed under with mortality trials, showing invariably a highly significant 10-30 % relative increase in survival. Mortality is considered an important endpoint, and this may be so. Yet, a relative increase in survival of 10-30 % generally means in absolute terms an increase of no more than 1-2 %. Mortality is an insensitive variable of the effects of preventive medicine that is begun when subjects are middle-aged. At such ages the background noise associated with senescence becomes high. The endpoints better be reduction in morbidity so far. In addition, many clinicians know that patients would prefer assessment of quality of life and reduced morbidity rather than 1-2 % increased survival in return for long term drug treatment with considerable side effects. Relative risk reductions are frequently overinterpreted by clinicians in terms of absolute risk reductions. And so are underpowered P-values: a P-value of 0.05 afterall means the chance of a type II error of 50%.

On the other hand, statistics can do a lot more for clinicians than calculating P-values and relative risk reductions. Multivariate analyses can be used not only for exploring new ideas, but also for increasing precision of point estimates in a trial. Benefit/risk analyses of trial data are helpful to provide relevant arguments for clinical decision making, and they are particularly so when their ratios is assessed quantitatively. Statistics can provide us with wonderful meta- analyses of independent trials to find out whether scientific findings are consistent and can be generalized across populations.

9.LIMITATIONS OF STATISTICS

Of course, we should avoid giving a non-stop laudatio of statistics only. It is time that we added a few remarks on its limitations and possible disadvantages in order to express a more balanced opinion. Statistics is at the interface of mathematics and biology. Therefore, it gives no certainties, only chances. What chances? E.g., chances that hypotheses are true or untrue. We generally reject the null-hypothesis of no effect at $P<0.05$. However, $P=0.05$ means 5% chance of a type I error of finding a difference where there is none, and 50% chance of a type II error of finding no difference where there is one. It pictures pretty well how limited statistical inferences can be. In addition to the risks of type I and type II errors, there is the issue of little clinical relevance in spite of statistically significant findings. A subanalysis of the SOLVD study[11] found no symptoms of angina pectoris in 85.3% of the patients on enalapril and in 82.5% of the patients on placebo (difference statistically significant at $P<0.001$). In situations like this, one has to wonder about the clinical relevance of the small difference. This is even more so when one considers that an active compound generally causes more side-effects than does a placebo. Finally, we have to consider the point of bias. Arguments have been raised that controlled clinical trials although they adjust for placebo effects and time effects, are still quite vulnerable to other biases, e.g., psychological biases and selection biases. In clinical trials, as opposed to regular patient care, patients are generally highly compliant; their high compliance is an important reason for participating in the trials in the first place. They have a positive attitude towards the trial and anticipate personal benefit from it, a mechanism which is known as the Hawthorne effect.[12] Alternatively, patients selected for a trial often refuse to comply with randomization which may render unrepresentative samples.[13] Statistics has great difficulty in handling such effects and is, essentially, unable to make sense of unrepresentative samples. Not being familiar with statistics raises a two-way risk: you're not only missing the benefit of it but also fail to adequately recognize the limitations of it.

10.CONCLUSIONS

1. Statistics is fun for the clinical investigator because it generally confirms or largely confirms his/her prior hypotheses.
2. Accounting some simple statistical principles can help the clinical investigator reduce imperfections in the design and execution of clinical trials.
3. For the clinical investigator getting a good command of non-classical study designs can provide worthwhile extras to his/her research.
4. Statistics is not like algebra, because it requires a lot of biological thinking and just a little bit of mathematics.
5. Statistical analyses can be readily performed on such modern quality of life assessments like general feeling of well-being, physical activity domains, psychosocial performance etc.
6. Along this line the art of medicine is more and more being turned into scientific evidence.
7. Statistics can do a lot for the clinical investigator if he/she intuitively knows what statistics can and what it cannot answer.
8. Statistics can help clinical investigators to interpret more adequately limitations as well as benefits of current clinical research.
9. Statistics has, of course, limitations of its own. It can not give certainties, only chances.
10. Statistical significance does not automatically indicate clinical relevance. Statistical methods can not test every possible source of bias in a trial.

Not being familiar with statistics raises a two-way risk: you're not only missing the benefit of it but also fail to adequately recognize its limitations. We hope that this book will be an incentive for readers to improve their statistical skills in order to better understand the statistical data as published in the literature and to be able to take better care of their own experimental data.

11. REFERENCES

1. SAS Statistical Software 2000 New York, NY, USA.
2. SPSS Statistical Software 2000 Chicago, IL, USA.
3. Cleophas TJ. Methods for improving drug trials. Clin Chem Lab Med 1999; 37: 1035-41.
4. Cleophas TJ, Zwinderman AH. Limits of randomized trials, proposed alternative designs. Clin Chem Lab Med 200; 38: 1217-23.
5. Farewell VT, Dángio GJ. Report of the National Wilms'Tumor Study Group. Biometrics 1981; 37: 169-76.
6. Sacks H, Chalmers TC, Smith H. Randomized versus historical controls for clinical trials. Am J Med 1982; 72: 233-40.
7. Pocock SJ 1988 Clinical trials. A practical approach. Wiley, New York, USA
8. Whitehead J 1998 Planning and Evaluating Sequential Trials (PEST, version 3). Reading: University of Reading (www.reading.ac.uk/mps/pest/pest.html)
9. Lauter J. Exact t and F-tests for analyzing studies with multiple endpoints. Biometrics 1996; 52: 964-70.
10. Medical Research Council. Streptomycin Treatment of pulmonary tuberculosis. Br Med J 1948; 2: 769 –82.
11. Yusuf S, Pepine CJ, Garces C. Effect of enalapril on myocardial infarction and angina pectoris in patients with low ejection fraction. Lancet 1992; 340: 1173-8.
12. Campbell JP, Maxey VA, Watson WA. Hawthorne effect: implications for prehospital research. Ann Emergency Med 1995; 26: 590-4.
13. Cleophas TJ. The use of a placebo-control group in clinical trials. Br J Clin Pharmacol 1997; 43: 219-21.

Appendix

T-Table: v= degrees of freedom for t-variable, Q=area under the curve right from the corresponding t-value, 2Q tests both right and left end of the total area under the curve

v	Q = 0.4 2Q = 0.8	0.25 0.5	0.1 0.2	0.05 0.1	0.025 0.05	0.01 0.02	0.005 0.01	0.001 0.002
1	0.325	1. 000	3.078	6.314	12.706	31.821	63.657	318.31
2	.289	0.816	1.886	2.920	4.303	6.965	9.925	22.326
3	.277	.765	1.638	2.353	3.182	4.547	5.841	10.213
4	.171	.741	1.533	2.132	2.776	3.747	4.604	7.173
5	0.267	0.727	1.476	2.015	2.571	3.365	4.032	5.893
6	.265	.718	1.440	1.943	2.447	3.143	3.707	5.208
7	.263	.711	1.415	1.895	2.365	2.998	3.499	4.785
8	.262	.706	1.397	1.860	2.306	2.896	3.355	4.501
9	.261	.703	1.383	1.833	2.262	2.821	3.250	4.297
10	0.261	0. 700	1.372	1.812	2.228	2.764	3.169	4.144
11	.269	.697	1.363	1.796	2.201	2.718	3.106	4.025
12	.269	.695	1.356	1.782	2.179	2.681	3.055	3.930
13	.259	.694	1.350	1.771	2.160	2.650	3.012	3.852
14	.258	.692	1.345	1.761	2.145	2.624	2.977	3.787
15	0.258	0.691	1.341	1.753	2.131	2.602	2.947	3.733
16	.258	.690	1.337	1.746	2.120	2.583	2.921	3.686
17	.257	.689	1.333	1.740	2.110	2.567	2.898	3.646
18	.257	688	1.330	1.734	2.101	2.552	2.878	3.610
19	.257	.688	1.328	1.729	2.093	2.539	2.861	3.579
20	0.257	0.687	1.325	1.725	2.086	2.528	2.845	3.552
21	.257	.686	1.323	1.721	2.080	2.518	2.831	3.527
22	.256	.686	1.321	1.717	2.074	2.508	2.819	3.505
23	.256	.685	1.319	1.714	2.069	2.600	2.807	3.485
24	.256	.685	1.318	1.711	2.064	2.492	2.797	3.467
25	0.256	0.684	1,316	1.708	2.060	2.485	2.787	3.450
26	.256	.654	1,315	1.706	2.056	2.479	2.779	3.435
27	.256	.684	1,314	1.701	2.052	2.473	2.771	3.421
28	.256	.683	1,313	1.701	2.048	2.467	2.763	3.408
29	.256	.683	1.311	1.699	2.045	2.462	2.756	3.396
30	0.256	0.683	1.310	1.697	2.042	2.457	2.750	3.385
40	.255	.681	1.303	1.684	2.021	2.423	2.704	3.307
60	.254	.679	1.296	1.671	2.000	2.390	2.660	3.232
120	.254	.677	1.289	1.658	1.950	2.358	2.617	3.160
∞	.253	.674	1.282	1.645	1.960	2.326	2.576	3.090

Chi-square distribution

	Two-tailed P-value			
df	0.10	0.05	0.01	0.001
1	2.706	3.841	6.635	10.827
2	4.605	5.991	9.210	13.815
3	6.251	7.815	11.345	16.266
4	7.779	9.488	13.277	18.466
5	9.236	11.070	15.086	20.515
6	10.645	12.592	16.812	22.457
7	12.017	14.067	18.475	24.321
8	13.362	15.507	20.090	26.124
9	14.684	16.919	21.666	27.877
10	15.987	18.307	23.209	29.588
11	17.275	19.675	24.725	31.264
12	18.549	21.026	26.217	32.909
13	19.812	22.362	27.688	34.527
14	21.064	23.685	29.141	36.124
15	22.307	24.996	30.578	37.698
16	23.542	26.296	32.000	39.252
17	24.769	27.587	33.409	40.791
18	25.989	28.869	34.805	42.312
19	27.204	30.144	36.191	43.819
20	28.412	31.410	37.566	45.314
21	29.615	32.671	38.932	46.796
22	30.813	33.924	40.289	48.268
23	32.007	35.172	41.638	49.728
24	33.196	36.415	42.980	51.179
25	34.382	37.652	44.314	52.619
26	35.563	38.885	45.642	54.051
27	36.741	40.113	46.963	55.475
28	37.916	41.337	48.278	56.892
29	39.087	42.557	49.588	58.301
30	40.256	43.773	50.892	59.702
40	51.805	55.758	63.691	73.403
50	63.167	67.505	76.154	86.660
60	74.397	79.082	88.379	99.608
70	85.527	90.531	100.43	112.32
80	96.578	101.88	112.33	124.84
90	107.57	113.15	124.12	137.21
100	118.50	124.34	135.81	149.45

F-distribution

df of denominator	2-tailed P-value	1-tailed P-value	Degrees of freedom (df) of the numerator												
			1	2	3	4	5	6	7	8	9	10	15	25	500
1	0.05	0.025	647.8	799.5	864.2	899.6	921.8	937.1	948.2	956.6	963.3	968.6	984.9	998.1	1017.0
1	0.10	0.05	161.4	199.5	215.7	224.6	230.2	234.0	236.8	238.9	240.5	241.9	245.9	249.3	254.1
2	0.05	0.025	38.51	39.00	39.17	39.25	39.30	39.33	39.36	39.37	39.39	39.40	39.43	39.46	39.50
2	0.10	0.05	18.51	19.00	19.16	19.25	19.30	19.33	19.35	19.37	19.38	19.40	19.43	19.46	19.49
3	0.05	0.025	17.44	16.04	15.44	15.10	14.88	14.73	14.62	14.54	14.47	14.42	14.25	14.12	13.91
3	0.10	0.05	10.13	9.55	9.28	9.12	9.01	8.94	8.89	8.85	8.81	8.79	8.70	8.63	8.53
4	0.05	0.025	12.22	10.65	9.98	9.60	9.36	9.20	9.07	8.98	8.90	8.84	8.66	8.50	8.27
4	0.10	0.05	7.71	6.94	6.59	6.39	6.26	6.16	6.09	6.04	6.00	5.96	5.86	5.77	5.64
5	0.05	0.025	10.01	8.43	7.76	7.39	7.15	6.98	6.85	6.76	6.68	6.62	6.43	6.27	6.03
5	0.10	0.05	6.61	5.79	5.41	5.19	5.05	4.95	4.88	4.82	4.77	4.74	4.62	4.52	4.37
6	0.05	0.025	8.81	7.26	6.60	6.23	5.99	5.82	5.70	5.60	5.52	5.46	5.27	5.11	4.86
6	0.10	0.05	5.99	5.14	4.76	4.53	4.39	4.28	4.21	4.15	4.10	4.06	3.94	3.83	3.68
7	0.05	0.025	8.07	6.54	5.89	5.52	5.29	5.12	4.99	4.90	4.82	4.76	4.57	4.40	4.16
7	0.10	0.05	5.59	4.74	4.35	4.12	3.97	3.87	3.79	3.73	3.68	3.64	3.51	3.40	3.24
8	0.05	0.025	7.57	6.06	5.42	5.05	4.82	4.65	4.53	4.43	4.36	4.30	4.10	3.94	3.68
8	0.10	0.05	5.32	4.46	4.07	3.84	3.69	3.58	3.50	3.44	3.39	3.35	3.22	3.11	2.94
9	0.05	0.025	7.21	5.71	5.08	4.72	4.48	4.32	4.20	4.10	4.03	3.96	3.77	3.60	3.35
9	0.10	0.05	5.12	4.26	3.86	3.63	3.48	3.37	3.29	3.23	3.18	3.14	3.01	2.89	2.72
10	0.05	0.025	6.94	5.46	4.83	4.47	4.24	4.07	3.95	3.85	3.78	3.72	3.52	3.35	3.09
10	0.10	0.05	4.96	4.10	3.71	3.48	3.33	3.22	3.14	3.07	3.02	2.98	2.85	2.73	2.55
15	0.05	0.025	6.20	4.77	4.15	3.80	3.58	3.41	3.29	3.20	3.12	3.06	2.86	2.69	2.41
15	0.10	0.05	4.54	3.68	3.29	3.06	2.90	2.79	2.71	2.64	2.59	2.54	2.40	2.28	2.08
20	0.05	0.025	5.87	4.46	3.86	3.51	3.29	3.13	3.01	2.91	2.84	2.77	2.57	2.40	2.10
20	0.10	0.05	4.35	3.49	3.10	2.87	2.71	2.60	2.51	2.45	2.39	2.35	2.20	2.07	1.86
30	0.05	0.025	5.57	4.18	3.59	3.25	3.03	2.87	2.75	2.65	2.57	2.51	2.31	2.12	1.81
30	0.10	0.05	4.17	3.32	2.92	2.69	2.53	2.42	2.33	2.27	2.21	2.16	2.01	1.88	1.64
50	0.05	0.025	5.34	3.97	3.39	3.05	2.83	2.67	2.55	2.46	2.38	2.32	2.11	1.92	1.57
50	0.10	0.05	4.03	3.18	2.79	2.56	2.40	2.29	2.20	2.13	2.07	2.03	1.87	1.73	1.46
100	0.05	0.025	5.18	3.83	3.25	2.92	2.70	2.54	2.42	2.32	2.24	2.18	1.97	1.77	1.38
100	0.10	0.05	3.94	3.09	2.70	2.46	2.31	2.19	2.10	2.03	1.97	1.93	1.77	1.62	1.31
1000	0.05	0.025	5.04	3.70	3.13	2.80	2.58	2.42	2.30	2.20	2.13	2.06	1.85	1.64	1.16
1000	0.10	0.05	3.85	3.00	2.61	2.38	2.22	2.11	2.02	1.95	1.89	1.84	1.68	1.52	1.13

Paired non-parametric test: Mann-Whitney test,
the table uses smaller of the two ranknumbers

N pairs	P<0.05	P<0.01
7	2	0
8	2	0
9	6	2
10	8	3
11	11	5
12	14	7
13	17	10
14	21	13
15	25	16
16	30	19

Unpaired non-parametric test: Wilcoxon rank sum test. Table uses difference of added up rank numbers between group 1 and group 2

P<0.01 levels

n_2 ↓ / n_1 →	2	3	4	5	6	7	8	9	10	11	12	13	14	15
4			10											
5		6	11	17										
6		7	12	18	26									
7		7	13	20	27	36								
8	3	8	14	21	29	38	49							
9	3	8	15	22	31	40	51	63						
10	3	9	15	23	32	42	53	65	78					
11	4	9	16	24	34	44	55	68	81	96				
12	4	10	17	26	35	46	58	71	85	99	115			
13	4	10	18	27	37	48	60	73	88	103	119	137		
14	4	11	19	28	38	50	63	76	91	106	123	141	160	
15	4	11	20	29	40	52	65	79	94	110	127	145	164	185
16	4	12	21	31	42	54	67	82	97	114	131	150	169	
17	5	12	21	32	43	56	70	84	100	117	135	154		
18	5	13	22	33	45	58	72	87	103	121	139			
19	5	13	23	34	46	60	74	90	107	124				
20	5	14	24	35	48	62	77	93	110					
21	6	14	25	37	50	64	79	95						
22	6	15	26	38	51	66	82							
23	6	15	27	39	53	68								
24	6	16	28	40	55									
25	6	16	28	42										
26	7	17	29											
27	7	17												
28	7													

Unpaired non-parametric test: Wilcoxon rank sum test. Table uses
difference of added up rank numbers between group 1 and group 2

P<0.05 levels

n_2 ↓ \ n_1 →	2	3	4	5	6	7	8	9	10	11	12	13	14	15
5				15										
6			10	16	23									
7			10	17	24	32								
8			11	17	25	34	43							
9		6	11	18	26	35	45	56						
10		6	12	19	27	37	47	58	71					
11		6	12	20	28	38	49	61	74	87				
12		7	13	21	30	40	51	63	76	90	106			
13		7	14	22	31	41	53	65	79	93	109	125		
14		7	14	22	32	43	54	67	81	96	112	129	147	
15		8	15	23	33	44	56	70	84	99	115	133	151	171
16		8	15	24	34	46	58	72	86	102	119	137	155	
17		8	16	25	36	47	60	74	89	105	122	140		
18		8	16	26	37	49	62	76	92	108	125			
19	3	9	17	27	38	50	64	78	94	111				
20	3	9	18	28	39	52	66	81	97					
21	3	9	18	29	40	53	68	83						
22	3	10	19	29	42	55	70							
23	3	10	19	30	43	57								
24	3	10	20	31	44									
25	3	11	20	32										
26	3	11	21											
27	4	11												
28	4													

INDEX

Printed in the United States
34347LVS00003B/26